Pischinger
Matrix and Matrix Regulation

Matrix and Matrix Regulation

**Basis
for a Holistic Theory
in Medicine**

by Prof. Alfred Pischinger †, MD

Edited by Prof. Hartmut Heine PhD
English translation by Norman Mac Lean MD

With 37 illustrations and 18 tables

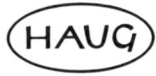

Editions HAUG INTERNATIONAL · Brussels

Pischinger, Alfred:
Matrix and Matrix Regulation. Basis for a Holistic Theory in Medicine / ed. by Hartmut Heine. – Brussels, Belgium : Editions HAUG INTERNATIONAL, 1991.
ISBN 2-8043-4000-7

Printing history: 1st–8th German edition 1975–1990

Copyright German edition © 1975 by Karl F. Haug Verlag GmbH & Co. · Heidelberg, Federal Republic of Germany
Copyright English edition © 1991 Editions HAUG INTERNATIONAL s.p.r.l. – Brussels, Belgium

All rights reserved (including those of translation into foreign languages). No part of this book may be reproduced in any form – by photoprint, microfilm, or any other means – nor transmitted or translated into a machine language without written permission from the publishers.
Toute reproduction, adaptation ou traduction intégrale ou partielle du présent ouvrage, sous la forme de texte imprimés, de microfilms, de photographies, de photocopies ou tout autre moyen, ainsi que la traduction ou la transmission en langage machine ne peuvent être réalisées sans l'autorisation écrite de l'éditeur.

Editions HAUG INTERNATIONAL
Chaussée de Ninove 1072
B-1080 Bruxelles/Brussels

Titel-No. 4000 · ISBN 2-8043-4000-7

Dépôt légal: Bibliothèque Royale de Belgique
n° D/1991/6159/01

Imprimé: Progressdruck GmbH, 6720 Speyer am Rhein
Federal Republic of Germany

Contents

Introduction 7

Foreword 11

Part One
The Structure and Function of the Ground Substance (Extracellular Matrix). 13
Paradigms in Medical Thinking (by *H. Heine*) 13
Functional Unit of the Cell and the Extracellular Space 14
The Extracellular Matrix as a Protein Regulatur ("Slag Phenomenon") 27
The Influence of Matrix Vesicles on Ground Regulation 29
Leukocytolysis 31
Regulation of Tumor Extracellular Matrix 42
Significance of Chronobiology 43
Topography of Extracellular Matrix Distribution 44
Structural Components of the Extracellular Matrix 45
    Glycosaminoglycans (GAGs) 45
    Sugars of the Cell Surface – the Glycocalyx 48
    Basement Membranes 51
    Proteoglycans (PGs) 52
    Proteoglycan Synthesis 55
    Functional Aspects of Ch-PG-Hyaluronic Acid Complexes 57
    Dermatan Sulfate-Proteoglycan 58
    Functional Aspects of Dermatan Sulfate-Proteoglycan 58
    Heparan Sulfate-Proteoglycan 59
    Functional Aspects 59
    Keratan Sulfate-Proteoglycan 60
    Functional Aspects 60
    Structural Glycoproteins 60
    Collagen 60
    Collagen Modification 62
    Functional Aspects 64
    Elastin 66
    Functional Aspects 67
    Network-forming Proteins 69
    Fibronectin 69
    Functional Aspects 70
    Laminin 72
    Chondronectin 73
    Energy flow in the Extracellular Matrix 73
    Sugars - Witnesses of Precellular Evolution? 77
Literature 79

Part Two
**The Ground System, Regulation and Regulatory
Disturbances in Rehabilitation Practice** (by *O. Bergsmann*) 83
Physiological Regulatory Requirements 84
    The Organism – A Network System 84
    The Regulatory Cycle 84
The Functional Elements 84
    Regulatory Quality and its Disturbance 87

Chronicity as a Biocybernetic Problem ... 89
   Observations in Chronic Pulmonary Tuberculosis ... 89
   Pathogenetic Investigations ... 89
   Therapeutic Results ... 90
The Pathogenetic Consequences ... 94
   The "Tip of the Iceberg" ... 95
   The "Base of the Iceberg" ... 104
   Regulatory Disintegration ... 108
   Minimal, Chronic, Lasting Stress
   (Focus, Disturbance Field, Stoerfeld) ... 109
Diagnostic Phenomena ... 110
Diagnostic Guidelines ... 110
   Colloid State ... 110
Projection Symptoms of Internal Organs ... 111
   Acupuncture and Meridians ... 111
   Somatotopes ... 112
   Perfusion ... 112
   Humoral Parameters and Leukocytes ... 112
   Muscle Activity ... 113
The Point: - the Window to the Ground System ... 113
   Morphology ... 113
Diagnostic Methods ... 125
   Palpation of Clinical Signs Caused by Reflexes ... 125
   Thermodiagnosis, Infrared Diagnosis ... 125
   Electrodiagnosis ... 126
Regulatory Therapy ... 128
Literature ... 130

Part Three
Therapeutic Consequences of Ground Regulation Research (by *F. Perger*) . 132
The Puncture Phenomenon ... 132
   Bioelectrical Events with the Puncture Phenomenon ... 140
   Puncture Phenomenon and Oxygen Saturation of the Blood ... 141
   Iodometry and the Puncture Phenomenon ... 143
   Totality of Regulation in the Puncture Phenomenon ... 144
Testing the Initial State and Autonomic Asymmetry ... 145
Extraneural Mechanism for Control of Defence Processes ... 164
Neural Therapy According to Huneke ... 174
Therapeutic Consequences of Ground Regulation Research ... 188
   Selection of Specific Drugs and Avoidance of Delayed Effects ... 189
   Rehabilitation of Defence Capacity ... 192
   Conservative Therapy to Relieve Stress on the Regulatory Cycles ... 193
   Elimination of Scar Disturbance Fields ... 197
   Relief of Silent Chronic Inflammation (Foci) ... 198
   Rehabilitating After-treatment ... 200
   Success and Failure in Regulatory Therapy ... 201
Literature ... 203

Index ... 217

Introduction

Experience shows that new, fundamental, findings in medicine only become the common property of medical practitioners years or decades after their development.

Scientific material that reveals linear-causal associations is understood and integrated more easily than material describing multidimensional functional associations.

The problem of today's medicine is that it sees the two ways of thinking as contradictory, instead of using them as possible complementary ways to acquire knowledge. The special successes in the fields of surgery, acute diseases, particularly infections, among others, are due to linear-causal, cause-effect thinking. To a significant extent it is based on *Virchow's* cellular pathology and *Newton's* classical physics. Hence, the double-blind, randomized trial is seen today as the decisive pathway to the understanding of medical processes.

However, it could not be ignored that chronic diseases, which have increased significantly in recent decades, lie beyond linear-causal thinking, as do their pathogenesis and treatment. This is a decisive point in long-term medicine.

Developments in the cybernetics (*Wiener* 1962) and the thermodynamics of open systems became useful signposts in this situation.

These developments indicate that biological systems do not show linearity, but are highly integrated and are subject to a biological vital flow equilibrium (*von Bertalanffy* 1952).

They exchange energy and material with their surroundings as "open systems".

In contrast to the classical, closed systems (mechanical, Newtonian), open systems show that when there is an influx of non-chaotic energy, this can spread suddenly through the entire system. The essential points in this are the transmission and dissemination of information.

Expansion of knowledge is to be expected from consideration of the cybernetic systems, which opened up the prospects from the monocausal to multidimensional events.

In 1975, *A. Pischinger*, the Professor of Histology and Embryology at the University of Vienna, presented his concepts about "The Ground Regulation System" in the first edition of this book, and also described the sounding board on which the reciprocal effects in the human organism take place.

Pischinger was a student of such important teachers as *H. Rabel*, the Nobel Prize winner *Loewi*, *Albert von Bethe*, and *William von Möllendorf*; with his first publications, "A report on the isoelectric point of histological elements as the cause of their variations in capacity to accept staining", and others, he became the founder of tissue histochemistry. Basically, he concerned himself with the communications that connective tissue power uses to spread itself over the entire organism.

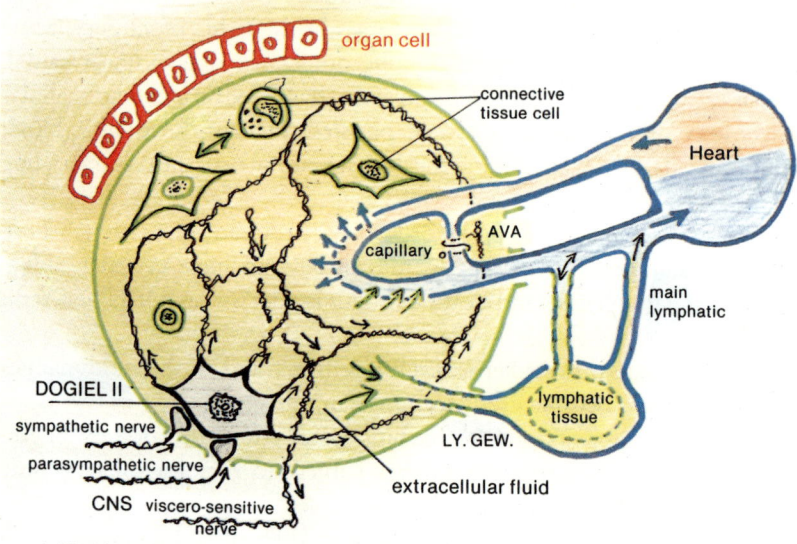

Fig. 1: The ground regulation system (historical scheme from 1960)

Today, *Pischinger's* system of ground regulation is defined as a function unit of the final vascular pathway, the connective tissue cells and the final vegetative-nervous structure. The entire field of activity and information of this triad is the extracellular fluid. The lymphatics and lymphatic organs are connected with it. It is the largest system penetrating the organism completely. It takes care of the nutrition of the cells (internal circulation) and the removal of waste products from them. Thus, it regulates the "cell milieu system" and is at the same time part of every inflammation and defence process. It is thus responsible for all basic vital functions.

All the organ cells depend on the intact function of the system for their existence; it guarantees the environment they need for survival. Organic diseases originate in dysfunctions of this system and its connections throughout the organism. The effects of a variety of noxious substances on the basic system (silent, chronic processes, heavy metals, the effects of stress, etc.), have been subject to observation in the Vienna School for four decades, using reaction measurement systems (*Bergsmann, Kellner, Perger*).

The dynamics of the functional processes (normal function, various dysfunctions, changes in the stimulation threshold) were measured on thousands of patients, using a variety of investigative systems. These showed a two-layer system in inflammation, and it was possible to classify this as being specific and non-specific.

The ground regulation system can react locally or generally. A variety of stimuli set off similar types of reaction in the non-specific part of the ground regulation system. *Hauss* and *Junge-Hülsing* from the Münster School arrived at the same results.

The Vienna School thanks effective and lasting successes in the treatment of chronic diseases to paying attention to the various individual stress factors in each patient, which support chronic illnesses, and knowledge of the reaction processes in the basic regulation system.

Examination and treatment methods were developed to bring about normalization of the functions of the basic system. In this way, chronic diseases which are regarded as difficult or impossible to treat (vegetative dysregulation, disseminated sclerosis, ulcerative colitis, rheumatic diseases, and, to some extent, cancer processes) became accessible to treatment. The cost-saving effects of this approach were confirmed impressively by *F. Perger*. Attention to the functioning processes in the basic regulation system opens up a genuine basis for prophylaxis.

Pischinger's system of basic regulation showed itself to be a teachable and applicable concept, encompassing all previous medical theory: humoral pathology, organic pathology, neuropathology, cell pathology and permeability pathology.

Gottfried Kellner, one of *Pischinger's* students, had a significant role in the development and formulation of this concept; his works have also been published in book form by Karl F. Haug Verlag.*)

---

*) Bergsmann, O., Bergsmann, R., Kellner, M. (editor): Grundsystem und Regulationsstörungen, Regulationspathologische Voraussetzungen für Diagnose und Therapie. Gedenkband für Prof. Dr. *G. Kellner*, Karl F. Haug Verlag, Heidelberg 1984.

Recently, three major schools have been active in the field of basic regulation, independent of one another;

1. *Pischinger* and his colleagues, who took over the tradition of the old humoral pathology according to *Paracelsus* and *Galen,* as well as, later, *v. Rockitansky* and *Eppinger.* The clinicians *Altmann, Bergsmann, Fleischhacker, Hopfer, Aiginger, Perger, Plohberger, v. Riccabona* and *Stacher* brought the theory of basic regulation into use in clinic and practice.

2. *Hauss* and *Junge-Hülsing,* University of Münster (universal mesenchymal reaction).

3. *Heine,* University of Witten/Herdecke.

With his fundamental research on the mesh structure of the matrix produced by the connective tissue cells, *Heine* has established the basis of informative reciprocal effects between cells, which can also be understood as applying to the entire organism.

After decades of experience with the basic regulation system which regulates the vital basis of all cells, it is becoming more and more clear that *Pischinger* was correct in speaking of a new basis for a total biological theory of medicine.

Bringing knowledge about the basic regulation system up to date made a completely new edition necessary.

Professor *Heine* took over the new arrangement of the book in cooperation with *Bergsmann* and *Perger,* physicians who are personally and scientifically close to *Pischinger.* This was only possible with the cooperation of the *Pischinger* family and the special interest of Karl F. Haug Publishers.

We are deeply grateful to them.

Cologne, Autumn 1988   Gisela Draczynski

Foreword

Current medicine is marked by the reductionistic principle of feedback of complicated natural processes (here, disease processes) on the interplay of simple parts of systems (here, syndromes). In this, it is overseen that the reductionistic principle only offers one way of looking at our real world.

For a long time, modern biology has recognized something which is only beginning to be accepted in medicine in our times, namely that all causal explanations of vital processes require a complementary explanation about the "sense and purpose" of both the parts and the functioning whole.

Alfred Pischinger's "Ground Regulation System" is interwoven with this thinking. His total biological theory of medicine is based on the concept that the causal explanation of the facts and their final explanation are not mutually exclusive, but complementary.

With the following contributions, the authors wish to pursue *Pischinger's* objects, and to indicate how important this complementary thinking is in the changing face of medicine. Bearing this in mind, the extensive revision of the previous edition can be understood.

Since it is generally agreed that one can only deal practically to the extent that one has a theory, the path adopted ought to be further revised through constructive criticism. That is our request to readers!

We thank Dr. *Ewald Fischer,* the publisher, who has not balked at venturing to support this new edition. We thank *Axel Treiber* from Karl F. Haug Publishers for his encouragement and rapid editorial work.

Herdecke, Autumn 1988   *Hartmut Heine*

Part One

The Structure and Function of the Ground Substance (Extracellular Matrix)

Paradigms in Medical Thinking

"Strictly speaking, the cell concept is only a morphological abstraction. Seen biologically, it cannot be accepted without the vital environment of the cell."

With these words, *Pischinger* (as late as 1983) perceived the weakness of the paradigm in *Virchow's* cell theory. In his work on cellular pathology, *Virchow* (1858) had limited the concept of disease to disturbances in the structure of individual cells. His basic concept is that each of the approximately 50 billion cells in the human organism is an "elementary organism", existing primarily for itself alone, enclosed and bounded by the cell membrane, but, incorporated in a working organism, playing its part in the function of the whole (*Frese* 1985).

The consequence of this linear cause-effect thinking, introduced into European natural science by *Galilei* (1564–1642), is that organisms are seen as complicated cellular functioning units, like technical machines, which, correspondingly, can be repaired when defects are present. In the end, it is only a matter of finding the disease-causing molecule in the cell. At present, it is believed that this has been observed in spot mutations in individual amino acids. This linearity in medical thinking has wide-reaching consequences in the therapy scheme of academic medicine; a drug has to attach itself to a suitable cellular receptor, and there can only be a reaction if the reactants fit together like a key in a lock.

In order to stick to a simple cause-effect relationship, this leads to being compelled to isolate the acute event from the intermeshed biological associations as a syndrome, and to treat it as such. "Particularly in chronic diseases and tumors, it is evident that the difference between effect and efficacy can scarcely be perceived" (*Fülgraff* 1985). This causal-analytical linearity thus has influence on the method theory of clinical trials and drug therapy. The individual phenomenon of being ill is subordinated to a type of disease. This is objectivized in a model, and thus becomes causal-analytically instrumentally accessible. Reality is replaced by models which have to be all the more reduced the more complex the reality. "To this extent, medical experience is not cultivated any more, since it is a question of models and not reality (*Fülgraff* 1985)." A model possesses neither the parameters for individual biological determinants nor for quality of life.

Since, additionally, a variety of diseases can be concealed behind the same symptoms, the randomized, double-blind clinical trial can only be one way of obtaining knowledge. It is undoubtedly wrong to stylize it as the only method, since casuistics and experience reports can do precisely that which the "objective" controlled clinical trial can not do: placing the individual in the foreground of medical attention, before the disease. The reason for *Virchow's* cellular paradigm being so successful in modern medicine is that particularly in acute diseases and those caused by microorganisms, there are individual causes that can be objectivized, and can be eliminated or repaired immediately. However, in the current situation of increasing chronic disease and tumors, this is hardly ever successful.

Functional Unit of the Cell and the Extracellular Space

Cells have a reciprocal relationship to their environment. Sea water is the primary regulation system of the single cell; the ion composition of the structured extracellular space of multicellular organisms corresponds to this. The milieu surrounding of a cell forms a structured basic substance in multicellular organisms (extracellular matrix), which has a significant effect on determining the genetic expressivity of a cell (*Hay* review 1983). Macroscopically, the organization of the extracellular matrix with connective and supporting tissues and blood can be visualized. The molecular biology concerns sugar polymers; either in free form, or in a variety of forms of protein and lipid binding, these form intercellular substances and the individual sugar surface film (glycocalyx) of a cell.

Bordeu (1767) had already arrived at the conclusion that connective tissue has more than a supporting and filling function, and that it has nutrition and regeneration tasks in the service of specific organ functions as well as in the the mediation of nerve and vascular functions.

C.B. Reichert (1845) also understood the connective tissue not only as a mechanically binding but organically vital(!) medium, and recognized that the nerves and vessels do not come into direct contact with the functioning cells at any point in the body, but that the connective tissue is the mediating member, the bearer of the nerve and nutrition flow, and that the reciprocal effects pass through it everywhere. Only the connective tissue has direct contact with all parts of the body. But there were no points of reference on the nature of the mediating action of the connective tissue.

Nevertheless, until very recently histological and biochemical techniques were not in a position to make a precise structural analysis of the basic substance. Cells, which were easier to record and comprehend, also fitted-in very well as a model of the smallest building bricks of an organism in the causal-analytical way of thinking at the beginning of the technical age.

Only now, with knowledge of cybernetic relationships and open energy systems, are we beginning to reconsider this overemphasized, positivistic point of view. It is of course true that warning was given at an early stage about a one-sided, model-type cell concept and the ignoring of humoral factors (*Rokitansky* 1846, *v. Rindfleisch* 1869, *Buttersack* 1912):

"It was a bold and useful thought of *Virchow's* to follow-up local disturbances down to the level of the individual cell; with this, *Virchow* freed pathology from the vagueness of *one-sided humoral* and *neuristic* concepts. But it went one step too far in the specification of the terrain. It is perfectly possible to recognize the individuality of cells and at the same time consider the structures that limit their functional and nutritional autonomy. Certainly, the cells of the parenchyma can be excited and be active, but in this connection they are partly dependent on the nervous system; they feed themselves and grow, but in this connection they are partly dependent on the vascular system. The terrain where local disturbances take place has three parts, parenchyma, capillary networks and nerve endings. However, we can not stay put at this. The anatomical composition of these parts is also subject to certain general rules, and here the connective tissue plays an outstanding role. *Connective tissue* inserts itself everywhere between the bloodstream and the principal structural parts. In doing this, it adjusts its histological transformation to the individual needs of the site in a wonderfully complete way. For our current purpose, the only position to be considered is that which the connective tissue adopts as a mediator between the parenchyma on the one side and its blood and nerve supply on the other. It is known that physiology has little to say about a *transmitter function* in the connective tissue. On the other hand, pathology has to pay attention to a whole series of apparently random points, whose cognizance is of great importance for understanding tissue alterations in disease. As regards nutrition via the blood, pathologists place great emphasis on the *capillary membrane* as an *endothelial limiting layer of the connective tissue(!),* and do not see the supply of the parenchyma with nutrition material as a general soaking and rinsing process, but as tied to a current of secretory juices that leaves the blood near the cementing borders that unite the rhombic endothelial cells into a closed membrane. Beyond the capillary membrane the current mainly continues through a network of juice canaliculi which is more or less sharply demarcated from the adjacent matrix of the connective tissue, and contains nuclei with dependent protoplasm remnants in its nodal points, the so-called connective tissue corpuscles. In this way the nutritional fluid penetrates up to the spaces enclosing the functioning parenchymal cells, and puts itself at their disposal. Afterwards, laden with regressive products from the metabolism of the parenchymal cells, it is taken up in the openings of the lymphatics, which are found abundantly in the connective tissue. In summary – everything that comes out of the blood takes a somewhat complicated route through the connective tissue to the parenchymal cells and then into the lymphatic system. When I look ahead and think about how often I will have to follow this path with my reader, and how every understanding of the local state of disease is tied to the stages of this path, I would like to tell him to take the perceptive route of pathological histology".

Buttersack arrives at the same point of view. His writings include, "that the layer that one has long called connective tissue is not simply a connecting material between the organs, that it does not simply carry-in and carry-out juices to form new parenchymal cells. It will become increasingly clear that if connective tissue is really a living part of the organism, all the attributes of life and all basic functions will have to be attributed to it." Thus, not simply a "transit route". In view of the situation, one has to agree with *Buttersack* in his finding the name "connective tissue" an unsuitable one for characterizing the nature of this tissue. It is, however, not easy to choose a suitable name. "Perhaps the word *basic tissue* comes near to what is sought. It has been known for a long time that the tissues in question form the basis of the entire body; but also in the figurative sense, it is the basis where all organs have their roots, and in the end it has, to a certain extent, its own basic, essential value *(Buttersack)."*

In *Ricker's* Relation Pathology (1924) and *Eppinger's* Permeability Pathology (1949) the functional connection between the capillary bed and the cell via the extracellular matrix, and its disturbances as the starting-point of many diseases, are also recognized. *Ricker* showed that many processes and events that are involved in healthy and pathological events in the body are nothing more than variations in one and the same basic physiological process. Variations in metabolism and energy exchange; variations of degree and site ("law of degrees"). With this, *Ricker* was able to confirm the experience medicine taught by *Hippocrates, Galen, Paracelsus* and *Hahnemann*, where all disease processes are of the same type, and that not the substance, but the dosage, is the healing factor; and hence many diseases could be healable with the healing dose of one and the same medication, and the healing dose of numerous medications could alleviate one and the same disease, or might be able to heal it, just as experience indicates.

All these above authors present observations and evidence that the "ground system" is primarily affected in every type of disease process, and that it plays a significant role in healing processes.

So this is the picture from the older literature: the connective tissue body with the cells, fibers and interfiber masses is accepted as a united complex that surrounds the specifically working parenchymal cells, and makes their maintenance and regeneration possible. This connective tissue body also can not be considered separately from the vessels, or capillaries, or from blood and its formation centers. Many new descriptions of alterations in the connective tissue, such as desmoses, collagenoses or geloses are thus, to this extent, misleading, as they always only consider *one* of the components of the connective tissue: either the fibers or the interfiber fluid. It should not go unrecognized that the cell is also the central point in the connective tissue. It, and its reactions, which have been known to pathologists for a long time, are the visible expression of the autonomous activity and reactive ability of the connective tissue.

The result was the retention of interest in the connective tissue. However, the work is more concerned with its physiological performance and biological tasks.

Prior to the victory of the *Virchow* cell theory, the individuality in a disease was seen as an alteration in the body juices. Ideas on this go back to archaic times. *Alkmaion, Galen, Hippocrates* and their students differentiated between four body juices: blood, mucus, yellow and black bile; their correct mixture (eukrasia) was the basis of health; a disturbed mixture (dyscrasia) was the basis of disease. The juices were seen as the bearers of the physical constitution. The humoral theory was built up into a major theory by a contemporary of *Virchow's,* the Viennese pathologist *v.Rokitansky,* but since humoral pathology at that time was not able to present the same firm evidence as *Virchow's* cellular pathology, it was put to one side in the years following. Only *Pischinger* and his co-workers, since 1945, have given the humoral theory a rational medical-scientific methodology as the basic regulation system. They have taken the cell isolated by *Virchow* out of its abstraction and placed it in the triad of the capillary, the basic substance and the cell, as the smallest common functional denominator of life in a vertebrate organism.

Cybernetics, which appeared at approximately the same time (*Wiener* 1963), and the development of the theory of *"Thermodynamic energy of open systems"* have shown that biological systems do not have linearity, but are highly intermeshed and are subject to a biological flow balance (*v.Bertalanffy* 1952). That is, biological systems are energetically open, and are thus in a position to exchange energy and material with their surroundings. However, the arrangements that appear are not stable. They swing away from a thermal balance, which generally does not permit a return to the initial state (but nervertheless stability may be achieved that is otherwise only the property of minerals, e.g. in genetic material). In contrast to the classical closed, so-called Newtonian systems, open systems show that when suitable energies are fed-in (non-chaotic energy, e.g. nutritional materials), they can spread suddenly through the entire system; this leads to the appearance of new structures in an autocatalytic way, and these can also develop further to a higher order.

Taking cybernetic associations into account makes it necessary to quit the firm ground of monocausal thinking. For the most part, no causal relationship is to be observed in biological processes between controlling input on the one hand, and the end results on the other (e.g. underestimated side-effects of drugs). "However, anyone who tries to apply one-dimensional causal chains to intermeshed systems can no longer lay claim to being scientific" (*Thomas* 1984).

The difficulties in finding linear cause-effect relationships in the organism are based on the fact that highly intermeshed energetic open systems are involved. The most suitable energy form to give a biological system structure and organization, and to maintain these, is information input and processing. The major significance of information as a non-chaotic energy form is that it is not tied to any particular energy carrier (e.g. sound waves in the air, information transmission by the auditory ossicles in the middle ear, further to the sensory cells in the cochlea, from there to the eighth cranial nerve, and finally transmission to the appropriate neuron areas in the brain). In the living system information is thus the most suitable energy carrier for setting-off both near and distant intercellular reciprocal effects (*Fischer* 1985). This corresponds to the aim of the organism to keep itself whole. It is certainly necessary to determine the individual conditions in a causal-analytical way, but with the increase in chronic diseases the conditions of a superior principle of order have to be sought, which serve as the basis for striving to maintain the organism.

This principle is given in the extracellular matrix and its regulatory mechanisms (*Pischinger* 1983). Correspondingly, the extracellular matrix permeates the extracellular spaces of the entire organism, reaches every cell, and always reacts uniformly. In epithelial cell groups or the brain, where the extracellular space is reduced to the minimum, the extracellular matrix forms the intercellular substance. Biochemically, the extracellular matrix forms a meshwork of high-polymer sugar-protein complexes, with the proteoglycans predominating (Figs. 1A, 1B, 2), followed by structural glycoproteins (collagen, elastin, fibronectin, laminin, among others). Proteoglycans (PGs), glycosaminoglycans (GAGs) and structural glycoproteins form a molecular sieve through which the entire metabolism of the capillaries to the cell and vice versa has to penetrate ("transit route"). Molecules over a certain size and/or charge are subject to an exclusion effect. The size of the pores in the filter is determined by the existing concentration of PG/GAGs in the tissue compartment concerned, their molecular weight, and by electrolytes and the resulting pH value. Here, the negative charge of the PG/GAGs has a decisive functional significance, which makes them capable of water binding and ion exchange of monovalent against bivalent cations.

They are thus the guarantors of isoionia, isoosmia and isotonia in the extracellular matrix (*Hauss* et al. 1968). The basic electrostatic tone established by this reacts to every change in the extracellular matrix with deviations in the potential. The information encoded in this way can inform the cell membrane as a potential deviation of the glycocalyx, and there, if it is strong enough (information selection!), lead to a cell reaction via depolarization of the cell membrane (e.g. muscle and nerve cells), or – as in all other cell types via activation of secondary messengers on the membrane (cyclic adenosine monophosphate, inosite triphosphate and many others) which transmit coded information in the basic substance to cytoplasmic enzymes. This lands in the cell nucleus and can finally come into contanct with the genetic material of the cell nucleus at the appropriate site. This is followed by transcription of the appropriate DNA part (gene) in the various types of RNA.

After transfer into the cytoplasm the various RNA types in the endoplasmic reticulum start translation of the information into products individual to the cell (Review by *Heine* and *Schaeg* 1979).

The mesh-type macromolecular superstructure of PG/GAGs plays an important role in the mechanical coherence of tissue (*Balasz* and *Gibbs* 1979, *Buddecke* 1971). Through this, the terminal axons of vegetative nerve fibers, for example, are subject to a specific mechanical and electrical tension, and can react with the release of neurotransmitter substances and neuropeptides. PG/GAGs form a shock-absorbing system that works like a lubricating substance (joint lubricant), which changes to a visco-elastic substance with severe and repeated mechanical demands. This is highly elastically malleable, and through this has an energy-consuming effect. The rheological changes thus also belong to the encoding of information in the ground substance (*Heine* and *Schaeg* 1979).

Since the extracellular matrix is connected to the endocrine gland system via the capillaries, and to the central nervous system via the peripheral vegetative nerve endings with their blind endings in the extracellular matrix, and both systems are connected to each other in the brain stem, superior regulatory centers can be influenced by the extracellular matrix. Since capillaries, vegetative nerve fibers and the connective tissue cells that wander through the connective tissue and regulate the extracellular matrix (macrophages, leukocytes, mast cells) are mutually "informative" through released cell products (prostaglandins, lymphokins, cytokins, proteases, protease inhibitors, etc.), the result is a vast, complex, intermeshed humoral system, whose historical scientific predecessors are to be found in the classical vital juice theory. The advantage of such an intermeshed system is

Fig. 1A: Reciprocal relationships (arrows) between capillaries (8), ground substance (matrix), (proteoglycans and structural glycoproteins 1, collagen 2, elastin 3), connective tissue cells (mast cell 4, defence cell 5, fibrocyte 6), terminal autonomic axons (7) and organic parenchymal cells (10). Basement membrane (9).
The fibrocyte (6) is the regulatory center of the ground substance. Only this type of cell is able to synthesize extracellular and nervous components. The main mediators and filters of information are the proteoglycans, structural glycoproteins and the cell suface sugar film (glycocalyx; dotted line on all the cells, collagen and elastin).

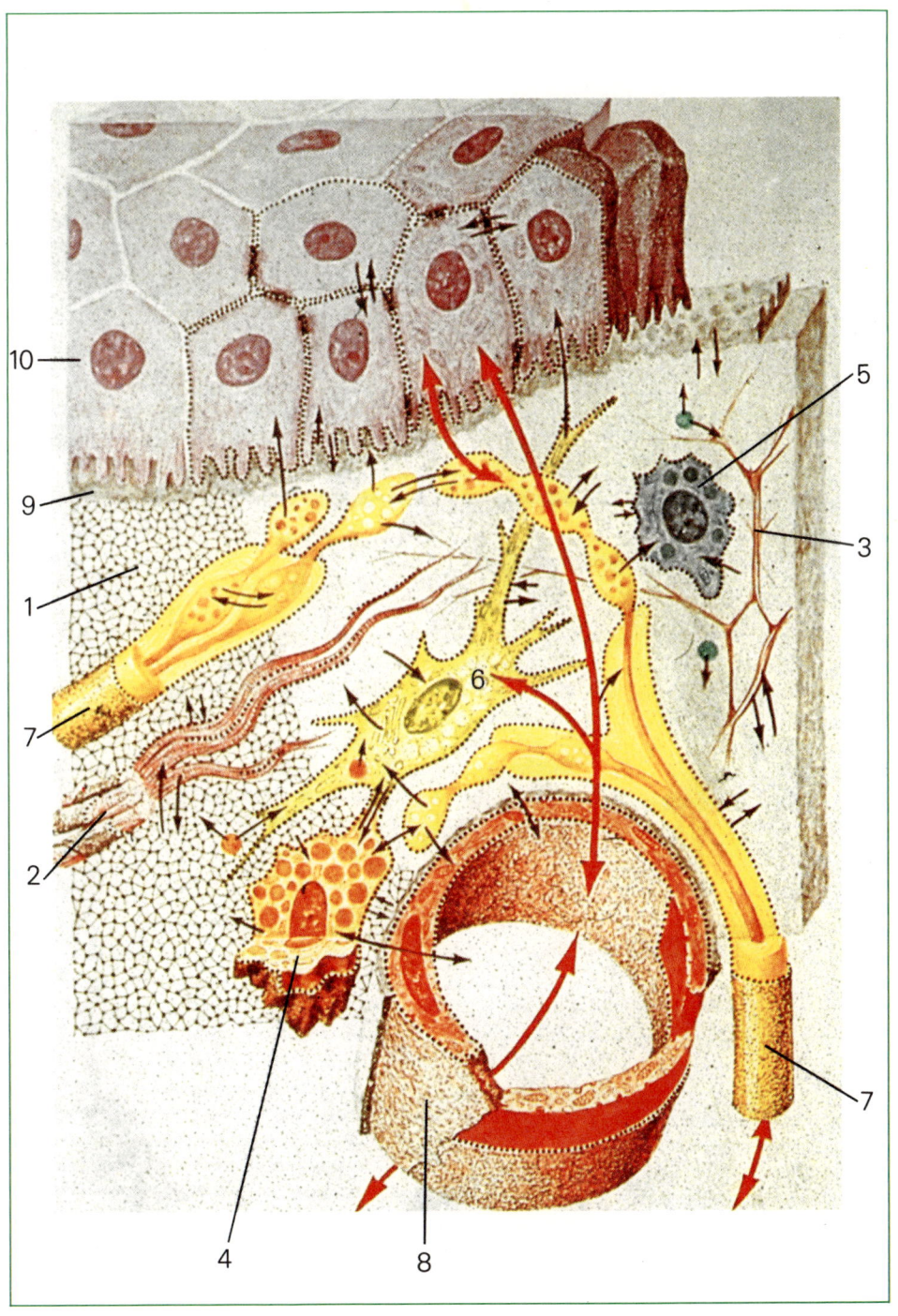

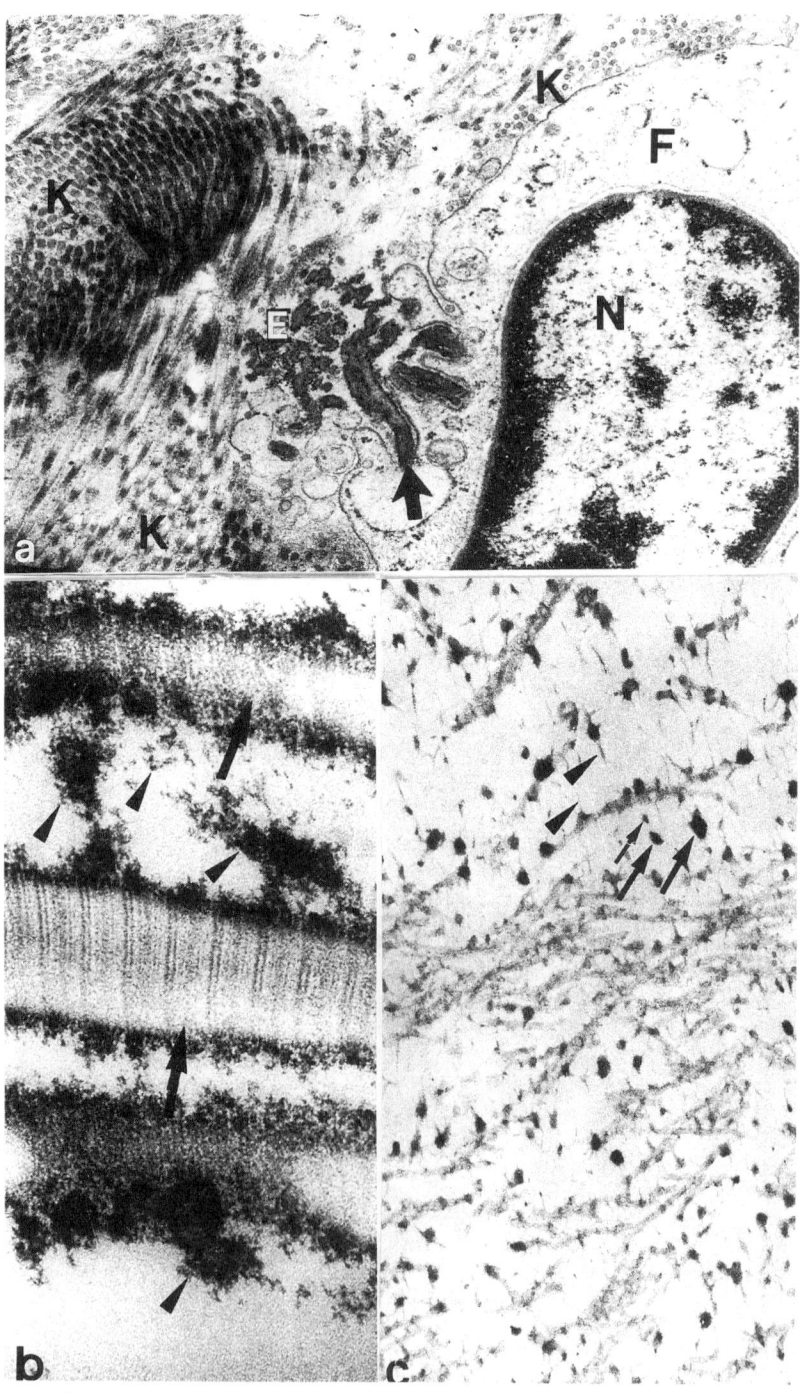

Fig. 1B: Ultrastructure of the extracellular matrix and matrix synthesis (cf. Fig. 1A). a) Skin (human). Section of extracellular matrix-synthesizing fibroblast F. The arrow indicates the extrusion of an elastic fibril. Collagen K and elastic fibrils in the extracellular matrix and on the cell surface. The proteoglycan network can be seen as a fine veil between the collagen fibrils. N = fibroblast nucleus. x 20,000. b) Skin (human). Striation of collagen fibrils (arrows) and the proteoglycans and glycosaminoglycans connected to the fibrils (arrowheads). The preparation was preincubated with ruthenium red (according to *Luft*) to show the sugars, and then fixed in osmic acid. Further treatment was conventional. x 75,000. c) cartilaginous extracellular matrix of a chicken at the 21st day of development. The extracellular matrix can be seen clearly. The electron-dense studs show the proteoglycans that have collapsed due to fixation (arrows) and the protruding arms the hyaluronic acid (arrowheads). x 56,000.

a significant increase in the adjustment and performance capacity, and the possibility of more and more properties that can not be attained through simple addition of the single properties of the components. In this way, relationships between the psyche and the immune system ("psychoneuroimmunology") can be understood (*Adler* 1981).

In spite of the higher specialization of sub-systems (e.g. the immune system), and the susceptibility associated with this, the evolutive value of highly intermeshed, biological systems lies in their overabundance. This means that "the system compensates for the failure of individual components or sub-systems by having other components or sub-systems being able to take over, completely or partially, long-term or short-term, until the defective components can be repaired" (*Thomas* 1984). Thus, the pur-

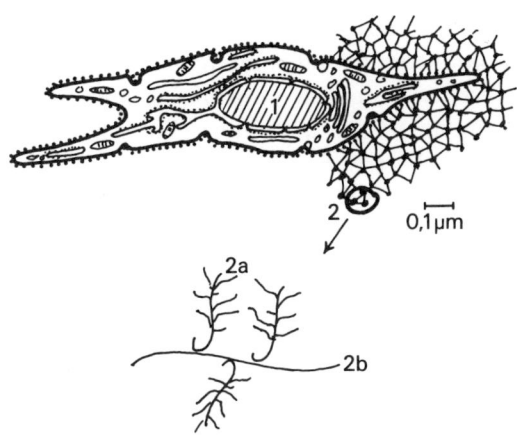

Fig. 2: Extract from Fig. 1A. Fibroblast (1) synthesizing extracellular matrix. The proteoglycan network pattern (2) is enlarged (arrow). Proteoglycans (2a) are bound to hyaluronic acid (2b) in the ground substance.

pose of steadfastness an organism towards maintaining itself is found in the regulation of homeostasis. In biology, as in medicine, causality and finality are thus not mutually exclusive, but are mutually involved.

Phylogenetically, the extracellular matrix is older than the nerve and hormone systems. In its formation and breakdown it is appropriately regulated by a very basic cell system in a compensatory way: the fibroblast-macrophage system. While fibroblasts are able to react to a situation within seconds with a quantitatively and qualitatively appropriate synthesis of proteoglycans and structural glycoproteins, macrophages, in the normal situation, can break down the extracellular matrix by phagocytosis. Since fibrocytes are not able to differentiate between "the good and the bad", the result in chronic alterations is the development of a extracellular matrix whose structure is not physiological, which can make an important contribution to the development of chronic diseases due to its influence on all the cellular elements (*Heine* 1972).

The sugar polymers of the extracellular matrix are thus suitable for information transmission and storage in the extracellular matrix due to their high water-binding and ion exchange capacity. This is different from the biopolymer DNA, which stores genetic codes; in the extracellular matrix it is not a question of information storage with the possibility of giving informatin further by transcription and translation, but of a rapidly arranged information transmission and distribution in the sense of actual regulation of homeostasis.

In my opinion, the structural combination of water and sugar biopolymers represents the oldest information and defence system of oxygen-breathing unicellular and multicellular living beings (in unicellular organisms as bacteria and viruses the sugar polymers are bound with the cell membrane at the external envelope). For these polymers are, in addition, suitable for helping the latent inflammatory readiness of the connective tissue to the level of homeostasis, as a redox system, through taking-up and giving-off electrons (*Levine* and *Kidd* 1985). Due to this redox system, every situation that alters the electrical tone of the extracellular matrix can be encoded, and reciprocally spread and processed throughout the organism. At the same time, excess extracellular electrons and protons in the form of oxygen and hydroxyl radicals, which appear in every enzyme-guided transformation, can be intercepted by the water and sugar polymers. The resulting heat is necessary for the further stimulation of biological processes. The regulatory capacity of the extracellular matrix thus has major significance in disease processes. In all acute and chronic diseases, including tumors, regulatory disturbances and changes in the ultrastructure can therefore be demonstrated (*Pischinger* and *Perger* 1983, *Heine* 1987).

In the course of evolution, the sugar polymers of the extracellular matrix experience a binding to the protein backbone, which leads to the term proteoglycans (an exception is hyaluronic acid; Figs. 2, 3, 4), or they are bound to the outer side of the cell membrane by membrane proteins (glycoproteins and glycolipids of the surface sugar film – the glycocalyx – the cell). All structural proteins (collagen, elastin, fibronectin, etc.) also experience glycosilation.

Sugars in the form of nucleotides are involved in most of the enzymatic reactions in the extracellular matrix and the cells, as part of

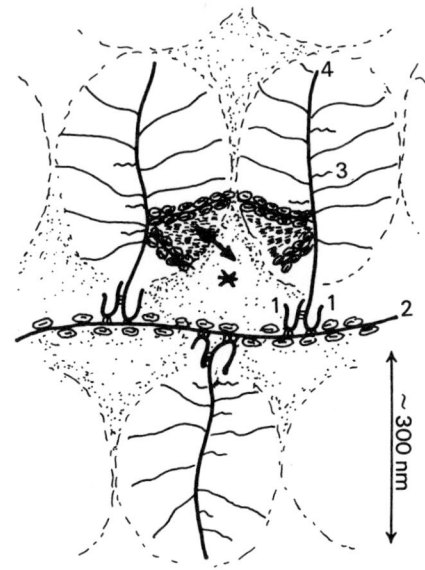

Fig. 3: Enlargement of Fig. 2. Link proteins (1), bind the proteoglycan molecules to hyaluronic acid (2). This is stretched due to its negative charge. The same situation exists with the polysaccharide chains (3), which are stretched away from the protein backbone. The interrupted lines give the "domain" of a proteoglycan molecule. The double arrow shows the liquid-crystal-bound water and the ion exchange capacity (arrow) between the polysaccharide chains.

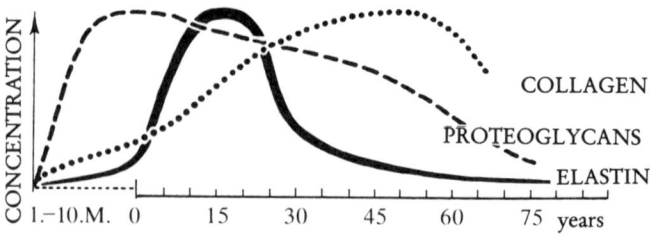

Fig. 4: Time-frame of the synthesis of the most important macromolecules in the extracellular matrix (proteoglycans, collagen, elastin). (after *B. Robert and L. Robert* 1974).

coenzymes. Nucleotides are built up from a base, a monosaccharide (almost always a ribose) and phosphoric acid. Precisely because coenzymes mediate between various enzymes, they have a special significance as a connecting link in metabolism, which is only possible for this reason. The term nucleotide indicates that this was first of all discovered as a building brick of the nucleic acids (DNA, RNA). Certain secondary messengers that mediate extra-intracellular information transfer, such as cAMP, cGMP and inositol phosphate contain a mononucleotide. An immemorial precellular evolutionary event seems to be reflected in this continuous "sugar principle of the living". The water-sugar biopolymers have always remained evolutively modern.

The Janus-facedness of this evolutive step became clear with the appearance of oxygen metabolization as the basis of life. On the one hand, the obtaining of energy from oxygen through the formation of ATP along the mitochondrial respiratory chain is necessary for more highly organized life-forms, and on the other, the resulting inflammation-promoting radicals have to be rendered harmless. The energy released in antioxidative enzymatic processes can be taken up by the water-sugar polymers of the extracellular matrix, which leads not only to a cooling of the "organisms reactor", but at the same time the energy needed for maintenance of homeostasis is made available. High energy electrons behave in a similar way, which, to a significant extent, originate from the oxidative breakdown of carbon-hydrogen bindings, as, for example in glucose breakdown (*Levine* and *Kidd* 1985). In the course of evolution important intracellular and extracellular antioxidant systems resulted such as intracellular superoxide dismutase, catalase, glutathion peroxidase, and, in the extracellular space, ascorbic acid, vitamins A and E, and many others. The electron and proton displacements that appear in enzymatic oxygen metabolism mainly lead to the formation of multiple radicals. Therefore energy is taken into the physiological redox potential of the organism via the ground substance. If the enzymatic stages responsible for electron and proton transfer are disturbed, which can begin focally, e.g. through inadequate blood supply, the result is an accumulation of radicals.

If this is long-lasting, the resulting non-pysiological alteration of the redox potential of the basic substance leads to the danger of the development of chronic inflammatory diseases, and even to the development of tumors (*Pischinger* 1983, *Perger* 1983).

The Extracellular Matrix as a Protein Regulator ("Slag Phenomenon")

Proteoglycans (PGs) are able to store all four nutritional substances; previously, too little attention was paid to this: carbohydrate as glucose and galactose, protein as NH groups, fat as carbohydrates with oxygen esters ("fatty acids") and water in the domain (deployment area) of PGs (*Wendt* and *Warning* 1986); water is the most important nutritional substance; when it is reduced in quantity, the brush-like shape of the PGs folds in and there is an adverse functional effect on the transit routes in the extracellular matrix (Figs. 1, 2, 3).

An important principle in currently valid nutritional theory is thus weakened: human beings do not have any protein stores other than fat cells, where excess calories are stored as triglyceride (*Rapoport* 1969). With more precise examination, one finds an increased quantity of collagen besides the fatt cells in the connective tissue of obese people (*Wendt* 1984). Since collagen fibrils need polysaccharides for side-to-side polymerization (overview in *Hay* 1984), these are also increased. Thus, protein can be stored in the form of collagen and proteoglycans. Thus, the entire ground substance of the organism has the capacity to be a protein store, with certain organs having preference.

Superfluous carbohydrates are stored in muscle and liver cells in the form of glycogen, but lead to an increased formation of PGs in the subcutaneous and interstitial connective tissue. That carbohydrate can be stored as PGs can also be confirmed by the finding that protein deposits on the basement membranes of capillaries and in the basic substance of diabetics have a higher sugar content than in non-diabetics (*Wendt* and *Warning* 1986). In addition, sugar can also be bound by non-enzymatic glyocolization of proteins (e.g. HbA_{1c}), collagen, elastin, proteoglycans, albumin, myelin, cell membranes, and many others. This reaction obviously has great significance in ageing processes, the genesis of arteriosclerosis and the tissue changes in diabetics (*Wendt* and *Warning* 1986, *Cerami* et al. 1987).

While the relationship of collagen to polysaccharide in stored protein is 95% to 5%, in pathological glycoproteins such as amyloid, the relationship is 42% collagen to 58% polysaccharide (*Wendt* 1984). Stored protein and amyloid, in differing quantities and combinations, can bind many other molecules ("slag") e.g. immunoglobulins, lipoproteins, fibrinogen-complement, albumin, amino acids, glycoproteins, defect- and foreign antigen proteins, uric acid, cholesterol, environmental noxious substances, carboxyhemoglobin. Hence, a protein storage disease is not necessarily of alimentary origin. The heteroproteins that arrive in the bloodstream are stored partly in the basement membranes and partly in the extracellular matrix. If the stored substances exceed the various individual capacities for breakdown, an increased shift to the transit routes takes place (such as inflammatory micro- and macroangiopathies, e.g. through carboxyhemoglobin deposits in the vessel walls in smokers, which can lead to intermittent claudication in the legs due to endarteriitis obliterans, or to death from a myocardial infarction due to coronary arteriitis [*Wendt* and *Warning* 1986]).

It is always a matter of deposits of metabolic waste ("slag"), which, for example, can be worked-off with protein fasting.

However, there are major individual differences in regeneration capacity, e.g. from the possibility of hydrolytic and proteolytic extracellular breakdown through lysosomes released from physiological neutrophil granulocytes or intracellular digestion by phagocytic macrophages.

The extent to which genetic and extracellular influences (disposition and exposition) cooperate here always has to be checked individually. A hint is given in Alzheimer's disease, which is accompanied by amyloid deposits in the brain. It has been shown that a precursor protein is involved in the formation of amyloid, and that it is coded on chromosome through a gene. Correspondingly, in Mongolism (Trisomia 21), there are amyloid accumulations in the brain in mid-life. There is a remarkable parallel between protein storage diseases and inherited familial hypercholesterinemia. In the last-mentioned, the LDL receptors are reduced in number, for genetic reasons, and there are mutations on the long arm of the 11th chromosome (*Hobbs* 1987). As a result, LDL molecules can only bind with a few liver cell receptors and thus be taken into the cells. The blood LDL level is correspondingly high, and with it the danger of arteriosclerotic changes. This is because cholesterol is the transport medium for LDL molecules, formed in the liver and depending on receptor-guided information. In spite of a high serum LDL level, the liver cells synthesize increased amounts of LDL-cholesterol as a supposed compensation.

The Influence of Matrix Vesicles on Ground Regulation

Only little observed, but still a physiologically and pathologically important regulation principle of the extracellular matrix, is the shedding of vesicular elements of connective tissue and defence cells in the extracellular matrix (*Heine* 1987a, 1988a, Figs. 5A, 5B). They disintegrate there under the release of a large number of biologically active substances that, apart from the vesicle contents (including proteolytic and hydrolytic enzymes and many cytokins), originate from the breakdown of the vesicle membranes (including prostaglandins and leukotriens).

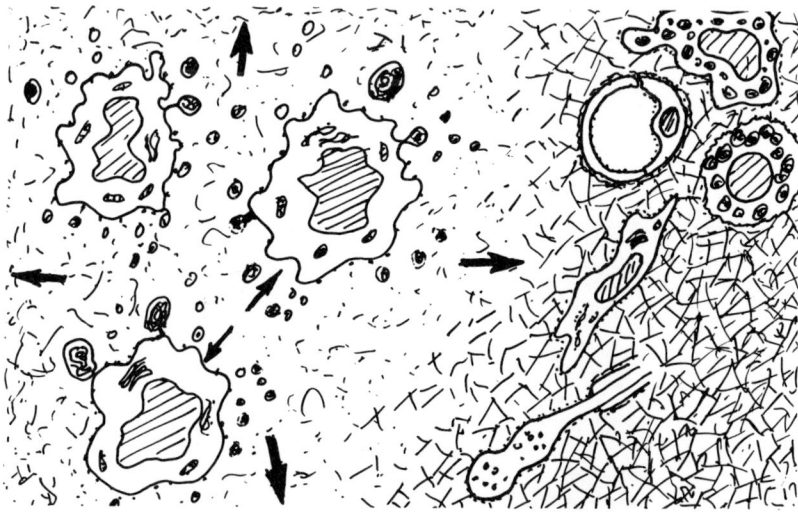

Fig. 5A: Regulation of tumor extracellular matrix by tumor matrix vesicles. In the left half of the picture there are 3 tumor cells with matrix vesicles being formed. The extracellular matrix has broken down into smaller fragments. The arrows show the spread of this principle into the surroundings as well as the mutual influence of the tumor cells on one another. The right side of the picture shows a normal extracellular matrix with typical cell components (cf. Fig. 1A).

Here, not only the pH value of the tissue is influenced, and with this an unspecific effect on the regulation of homeostasis, but also, in a similar way to individual glands in the autocrine (self influencing) and paracrine (related to their environment), cellular and nervous function is influenced (*Heine* 1987a, 1988). The phenomenon of physiological lysis of leukocytes described by *Pischinger* (1957) and *Kellner* (1975) also belongs to extra-

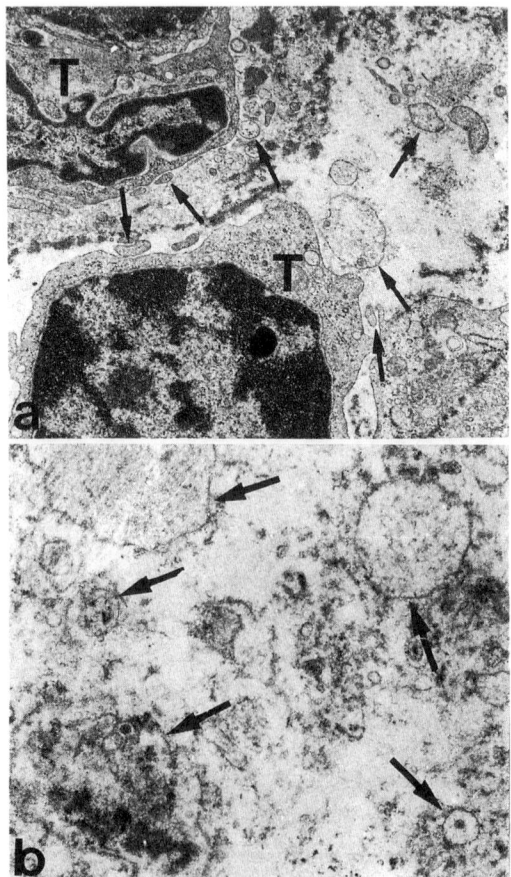

Fig. 5B: Scirrhous breast carcinoma. a) Formation of tumor matrix vesicles (arrows) on the surface of tumor cells /. x 5,000. b) Degenerating tumor matrix vesicles in the tumor extracellular matrix (arrows). x 7,500.

cellular matrix regulation. The enormous quantity of cytokins, lymphokins and tissue hormones released in this process is extremely suitable for the highly intermeshed system of the extracellular matrix to make an effect felt at many sites, in many ways, and simultaneously. Of necessity, this has to take place in an unspecific way, since the self-healing powers of the organism can be stimulated in a suitable way. The turntable of all natural healing processes and regulatory medical processes is thus the physiological lysis capability of the leukocytes (*Heine* 1988c). *Pischinger* (1957) brought this phenomenon out of oblivion when he sought an explanation for the phenomenon of why more leukocytes than the total quantitiy available in the blood enter the blood within 24 hours. In human beings this is by a factor of about 6 without any change in the figures in the differential blood count. *Pischinger* (1957) saw the cause in this way, "that up to now no attention has been paid to an important moment, namely the consumption of leukocytes in the blood".

Leukocytolysis

Pischinger (1983):
"The question of the *destiny of the leukocytes* has occupied hematologists for a long time, especially since *Undritz* described leukocytes in smears of native blood of healthy human beings and animals, which he interpreted as breakdown cells. These vary in size (7 to 24 microns). The cytoplasm is uniformly basophilic, and only contains an oxyphilic halo around the cell nucleus. The nucleus is completely structureless, pyknotic and mainly dark in color. Sometimes there is cell fragmentation. There are such breakdown cells for all the leukocyte types in the blood. However, they are very rare. *Koch, Heilmeyer, Laves* and others make similar statements (litarature in *Pischinger* 1957).

Later authors expose the blood sample to the effects of hypotension in vitro before making the smears (*Achard, Mauriac, Sampson, Storti, Schröder* and co-workers, among others). Here, various progressive forms of decomposition appear. Thus, this method is a genuine *resistance test* for the cells. *H.J. Schröder* presents not only relevant literature on the subject, but also a large number of personal investigations on the extent as to which leukocyte resistance can be influenced by physical, chemical, pharmacological and clinical factors. Depending on individual susceptibility, various degrees and types of swelling are produced.

In 1957, in an extensive paper on the fate of the leukocytes in the blood, I showed that decompensation forms are also found in the smears without prior forms of stress, which are generally similar to those appearing in hypotension as regards form and relative numbers. However, I do not believe that such cell remnants can be identified with *Undritz's* breakdown cells.

The following chapter is concerned less with the appearance of leukocytolysis as such, but more with the problem of whether and what relationships exist between leukocyte breakdown in the blood and the basic regulation of the organism; namely, whether the process can be regarded as a cell-milieu reaction.

In the paper on the fate of the leukocytes already mentioned, I was able to show that the absolute number of leukocytes in the blood in the rabbit ear reduces between artery and vein by an average of 17% (error probability p less than 0.001). Explanation of this needed precise analysis of normal capillary blood smears which were prepared with special precautions. I found breakdown products of all leukocytes in all stages, which had the same form as *Schröder* describes after the influence of hypotension; from naked nuclei to reticular and flat-shaped products, which only confirmed their origin from the cell nucleus through a positive Feulgen reaction, namely as nuclear material. I have therefore no doubt that there is a constant wearing-out of white blood cells. The extent of *"leukolysis"*, as I have termed the phenomenon, should now be investigated. Prior to this, the special smear technique has to be described, which avoids the appearance of exogenous artefacts, such as crushing.

It is best to make the smears with the edge of a 26 mm wide slide. The edge is specially prepared: the middle part is rubbed-down with abrasive paper (glued to an even base) to a width of 18–20 mm until there is a gap of about 1/10 to 1/20 mm when the smearing edge lies on the unabraded edges of the smear slide. With an angle of 25° to 30° between the two glass surfaces, the blood droplet – not too large – is spread along at moderate speed. Fast work is needed between taking up the blood droplet and making the smear, to avoid clumping the leukocytes at the edge of the blood film. Naturally, the blood should not come out over the edges of the rubbed-down part. In a preparation made in this way, the erythrocytes should be distributed in a simple layer, and the leukocytes (almost) evenly distributed.

Normal smearing equipment is not suitable for this: 1. the smear is too thick, due to the large angle of 45°, and 2. too much time is needed to make the smear, which means that the bulk of the leukocytes are found at the edges; 3. the fluting, which avoids crushing is difficult to apply to the slide.

The mechanical stress to the cells in the smeared blood droplet is the viscosity of the plasma. I described and analyzed preparations made in this way in the paper already mentioned, "The fate of the leukocytes", from different circulatory areas. In every smear of this type there is leukocytic lysis. The number varies according to the part of the body where the blood sample is taken, and the condition of the person investigated.

According to observations made by *Kellner* (personal information) on the behaviour of leukocytes with the addition of vitamin C in vitro, the destruction of the cells is at first unremarkable, but then sudden. One sees pale-stained, apparently swollen leukocytes in blood smears from small animals (guinea pigs, rats, mice), doubtless the first morphological signs of the beginning of lysis, which can also be recognized in the dark field. All these appearances simply can not be artefacts. Incidentally, I also emphasized at the time (1942) that a critically assessed "artefact" can have something biological to say. For example, if a smear shows *a Feulgen positive lysis form* close beside a *completely intact lymphocyte*, this means that they both must have been in *different states* because they were exposed to the same mechanical stresses.

It seemed sensible and useful to include the lysis forms of the leukocytes in the differentiation of the blood picture, to establish the extent of leukolysis. In apparently healthy people there are 5–7% lysis forms in blood from the finger pulp. With a 5,000 absolute number of leukocytes, there are about 300 lysis forms per mm^3; this means that if there is an even distribution through the body and 5 liter of blood, there are always 1–2 billion leukocytes in the process of decomposition. How many actually disappear completely can not be established by direct methods, as the duration of time between the beginning of the lysis process to complete disappearance of the cell is not known. However, it is possible to work out how many are decomposed in a unit of time from the extent of lymphocyte influx, under the assumption that they only disappear from the blood by lysis. With 25% lymphocyte and 5,000 total leukocytes there are 1,250 lymphocytes per mm^3; in a total blood volume of 5 l there are 1,250,000,000 x 5 = 6,250,000,000 = 6.25 x 10^9, namely about 6 *billion* lymphocytes. According to the literature – I have not investigated this personally – there is an inflow of about 6 time this amount, which gives 36 billion lymph cells. Thus, 36 billion have to *disappear from the blood* for the numbers to remain constant: 30 billion every 24 hours; that is 1.25 billion per hour, or about 20 million per minute, or 0.3 million per second. This figure is only valid for lymphocytes. Taking the 25% lymphocytes as a basis, the total number of leukocytes that disappear can be estimated at 4 times this amount, namely 1.2 million per second. If one now bears in mind that the smear only shows pre-stages, namely elements that are already affected, the relationship of 1–2 billion *in the stages of decomposition* to 1.2 million *cells that have actually disappeared* per second seems not to be improbable.

Little attention is paid to the facts described in today's clinical and theoretical medicine.

The first question is, *what significance do these appearances and processes have for the organism*.They possibly serve the maintenance of blood availability and supply. One only has to consider that leukocyte disintegration releases protein, amino acid produts, polysaccharides, lipids, nucleic acid, all sorts of tissue hormones and physico-chemical, oxidoreductive and surface-active complexes (*Pischinger* 1957). The UV spectrogram of methanol extracts of leukocytes, and also of fibroblasts, shows, for example, a specific color band in the same wavelength as our monocyte factor from blood. It is therefore not surprising that the investigatons by *G. Kellner,* described previously, show that the substances in the fibroblasts arriving for breakdown are able to influence the milieu, and how they do this. In both cases, leukocytes and fibroblasts, it is a matter of non-degenerating elements, namely *not the types with pyknotic nuclei,* which serve to explain the breakdown of the leukocytes *(Laves, Biermann).*

Systematic counting of the disintegration types in smears of many people in various conditions shows that the relative and absolute numbers per mm^3 (finger pulp) blood can vary a great deal. The next task has to be to explain the cause and significance of these variations. However, first of all, something has to be said about my counting technique: for reasons of precision I have always drawn blood up to the 1.0 mark (dilution 1:10), and counted all 9 mm squares in the Bürker's chamber. Counting a sample ten times with this method gives a standard deviation S = rounded up = 6%. The standard deviation of the mean runs at s_x = around 2%. Naturally, I always used the same combination of chamber and pipette in comparative counting. When necessary I used double measurements with two sets of equipment. The mean value gave the result. The single values were only used when they did not deviate significantly from one another by more than referring to the difference between the two counting chambers. Otherwise, the counting was repeated.

Some tables follow on the question of the behaviour of leukocytes (DBB) and lysis forms when the organism is influenced with monocytogenous serum remnant factor "M", and with penicillin. I show the DBB values in detail in order to show that the figures for all types of leukocytes change, as is known in hematology, and was shown specially by *Lickint* and also by *Storck* for short-term reactions, e.g. in radiation, hydrotherapy, hydrothermotherapy, douching, electrotherapy, etc. It is also known that the relationships in the lysis types also change under these types of influences (Lit., see *Schröder*, 1959).

First of all there is an example in the effect of an ml of Elpimed (Gebro = M 1:100). This corresponds to a dry quantity of about 100 micrograms (Tab. 8.1). As a control, the same subject receives 1 ml normal saline subcutaneously (Tab. 8.2) G. P., m., 15 yrs., 53 kg., hypertrophic tonsils.

Three examples from medical practice follow, where the known varying effects of monocyte factor and normal saline are checked further.

A final investigation with guinea pigs checks whether other influences can be differentiated from one another.

Three animals were used in the investigation, with approximately the same weight of 500 g, from the same litter of a pure strain.

The difference between the values in Tabs, 1,2,5 and 6 on the one hand, and Tabs. 2 and 7 on the other is seen clearly. The injection of *normal saline* in cases 2 and 7 produces *hardly any* changes worth mentioning in the leukocytes and lysis numbers. The minor variations, so far as they are not in the error area, can be explained by the fact that *a normal saline solution can only be physiological in relationship to the osmotic conditions, but does not correspond to the tissue as regards chemical conditions*, and this causes a modification of the milieu.

In contrast, subcutaneous injection of a ml of 1:100 dilution of active serum extract factor "M", diluted in normal saline (corresponding, as already said, to a dry quantity of approximately 100 micrograms of active substance) brings about a marked *increase in lysis forms* in both human beings and guinea pigs: in 1, for example, these increase from 325 to 382, 550, 1051 and 2720 in 9 hours, followed by a reduction to 646 the next morning (24 hour value).

Examples 3,5 and 7, as well as Table 8, show a major increase in the number of lysis forms in the hours following subcutaneous injection of 1 ml active serum extract (in 1:100 dilution), with a reduction in the lymphocyte count, as in example 1.

In example 4, on the other hand, the reaction to giving active extract "M" is absent: the lysis forms tend more to reduce in number, and the lymphocytes to increase. This reaction is thus the opposite of that in 3, 5 and 6.

This inverse reaction, which is not unusual (also in other areas), and the findings after giving penicillin (Tab. 8), are of special interest in the assessment of leukocyte appearances. In case 4, under the same influence as in the previous examples, namely giving active serum extract "M", the number of lysis forms remains high and the lymphocyte count increased. The cause for this can be sought in the *state of the organism*, and the field of activity of monocyte-promoting (active) serum extract "M". In fact, the subject in Tab. 4 had foci that have an adverse effect on the basic autonomic functions, according to our experience.

Example 8 also stands out. The animal died 3 days after a subcutaneous injection of 4,000 I.U. Na penicillin. The "toxicity" of *penicillin* in guinea pigs is known, but no clear explanation for this can be given. Damage to the intestinal flora is considered a possible cause. However, in our experiment, it is noticeable that the number of lysis forms *falls* significantly from 690 to 419 in 24 hours, as do the lymphocyte and eosinophil counts. In subcutaneous injection, the toxicity of penicillin for the guinea pig expresses itself in an adverse influence on the regulation of the blood. At the moment, more can not be said. It would be worth investigating whether the same takes place in human beings. In any case, *F. Perger* has established

Tab. 1

Time		Total No.	N	E	M	L	No.
5.1.	9.10	6490	2596	260	390	2920	325
	9.15	Injection 1 ml ELPIMED (Gebro)					
	9.35	6390	2860	254	254	2610	382
	10.00	5490	2910	220	275	1535	550
	10.45	4780	1720	240	287	1482	1051
	17.15	9380	3845	565	375	1875	2720
6.1	8.00	5380	2045	270	323	2100	646

Tab. 2

Time		Total No.	N	E	M	L	No.
12.1.	8.30	4780	1770	286	286	1960	478
	8.37	Subcut. inj. 1 ccm normal saline					
	8.57	5510	2315	220	275	2480	220
	9.22	4530	1721	408	317	1676	408
	10.07	4620	2217	277	416	1340	370
	16.37	6330	3165	253	443	1962	507
13.1	7.30	5600	2130	336	392	2350	392

Tab. 3

M. K., f., 50 y.: cephalic

Time		Total No.	N	E	B	M	L	No.
8.2.	9.00	5200	2288	208	104	104	2288	208
	9.05	Subcut. inj. 1 ml ELPIMED						
	10.00	5100	2400	408	0	102	1834	356
	12.00	5000	1650	300	0	300	1950	800

Tab. 4

H. P., f., veget. dystonia foci, extensive op. scars

Time		Total No.	N	E	B	M	L	No.
8.2.	9.00	3700	1665	74	37	74	1665	185
	9.05	Subcut. inj. 1 ml ELPIMED						
	10.00	3950	2014	79	0	158	1620	79
	11.00	4500	1845	45	45	180	2205	180

Tab. 5

R. P., m., 50 y., Vitium

Time		Total No.	N	E	B	M	L	No.
29.1.	8.20	4910	1720	245	0	440	2360	145
	8.25	Subcut. inj. 1 ml ELPIMED						
	9.20	4420	2080	221	0	486	1500	133
	12.20	5470	2740	95	0	383	1740	512

Tab. 6
Guinea pig., m., ELPIMED

Time		Total No.	N	E	M	L	No.
20.1.	9.15	10728	1952	867	217	6825	867
	9.25	Subcut. inj. 0,2/400 g KG					
	10.55	9640	3376	771	771	3180	1542
	16.55	8006	1865	648	466	3730	1297
21.1	8.30	7900	1658	632	475	4110	1025

Tab. 7
Guinea pig., m., Normal saline

Time		Total No.	N	E	M	L	No.
27.1.	10	7670	1189	1880	153	4065	384
	10	Subcut. inj. 0,2/400 g KG					
	10	6220	1120	1896	62	2550	497
	11	7100	1562	2200	71	2800	497
	16	7300	1533	2260	146	2810	438
28.1.	9	7840	1255	2038	157	4000	392

Tab. 8
Guinea pig., m., Na-penicillin

Time		Total No.	N	E	M	L	No.
3.2.	9	11439	2860	2630	343	4916	690
	9	Injection 4000 I.U. penicillin in 0,2 ccm normal saline					
	10	12022	1800	2650	120	6730	722
	16	5478	1646	930	220	2080	602
4.2.	8	8267	4962	992	413	1490	410

5 to 6 major reduction of lymphocytes and lysis forms

that penicillin reduces the serum calcium level in humans, although there is no "toxic" effect. However, sensitivity to penicillin has to be seen as a *regulation disturbance*, and, in this sense, an inhibition of regulation.

Consideration of leukocytolysis or leukolysis can not be regarded as final without taking into account 2 phenomena that are reported in the literature into account. These are: *Freund-Kaminer's cytolysis* and the testing possibilities with *Pichlmayer's* antilymphocyte or antigranulocyte serum; *H. Schröder* and co-workers report on this.

First of all, the *Schröder* investigations and the associated literature from earlier times should be dealt with, because they are freely connected with findings mentioned above.

Schröder's preparation concerns a standard osmotic treatment of the blood in vitro, which shows a variety of lysis forms, depending on the susceptibility of the leukocytes. Other authors used differing treatments, e.g. uric acid and salt with a small addition of oxalate (*Achard* and *Feuillie*). However, basically, natural blood smears from humans and animals were studied (*Undritz, Koch*), and the techniques used were more or less the same as those in the analyses described here. The same destruction forms are found in natural blood and treated blood.

Certain phenomena deserve to be emphasized in connection with the existing studies: after investigations with all the methods mentioned, the number of *breakdown cells can be influenced by drugs, and they are dose-dependent*. However, the most important points appear to be *Koch's* conclusions, drawn from investigations on natural blood: in his opinion, a "direct effect of the substance is not concerned in the various reactions, but the behaviour of the breakdown cells should be considered to be a *non-specific reaction*". In favour of this is the fact that many different types of procedures are accompanied by an increase in the number of breakdown cells, namely an increase in leukocytolysis. In *Koch's* opinion, there is possibly a specific endogenous active substance which might be formed in every case of an increase in the number of breakdown cells, from a variety of causes. This last conclusion brings us to thinking about the results of our own research. According to my experience, it could be a matter of the substances in the active serum extract; they are present in varying quantities, and normally *increase the lysis figures*. However, there must obviously be other factors with an inhibitory effect on leukocytes, as in the case of penicillin in guinea pigs. I also believe that this is not a matter of specific substances. The physical and chemical activities that the respective substances possess have corresponding effects. This means that we are dealing with non-specific processes.

The observations made by *J. Schröders* (1970) on the "Resistance test as an in-vitro method of determining the effects of antilymphytocytic and antigranulocytic sera" deserve special interest (ALS according to *Pischlmayr* and co-workers). Here, the immunosuppressive lymphocyte reactions that are decisive today for organ transplantation are connected to the field of non-specific regulation. Using original *Pischlmayr* antisera, *J. Schröder* was able to show that the efficacy and strength of ALS can be tested with resistance measurements on white blood cells. If this is the case, the antilymphocytic and antigranulocytic reactions must also have a root in the non-specific process. In general, that can also be understood: *for when the basis of vital functions fails, the specific processes can also not take their course uneventfully.*

The *cytolytic reaction* according to *Freund* and *Kaminer* (1919) also has to be dealt with in connection with leukocytolysis. It can make a contribution to understanding the process of cell lysis.

It is well-known that *Freund* and his co-worker *Kaminer* discovered that the serum of carcinoma patients has lost the capacity to break down cancer cells, which is present in healthy people. Later, it was shown that liver cells are also suitable for the test; but the hope that a cancer test had been discovered was not realized. The reason is that a loss of cytolytic capacity is also found in other serious diseases. For this reason, the use of the method as a tumor diagnostic system was judged more cautiously than initially. The phenomenon as such remained, however, an object of research. One speaks of cytolysins in normal serum, whose effects are inhibited in sick people. Here, the statement by Stern and Wilhelm is particularly important, namely that absence of cytolytic capacity is accompanied by damage to the RES. They believe that one of the tasks of the RES is to guarantee the normal lytic behaviour of the serum; for *loading the RES with dye causes the loss of the lytic function of the serum (rabbit experiments).*

In connection with these research results, we have to refer back to the works of *G. Kellner,* which have already been described in detail, on the cell-milieu reaction in cell cultures with alterations in the chemical and physical constitution of the culture liquid. It was shown that if the properties of the latter were not properly adjusted, there is massive cytolysis, and only then, obviously when the milieu is adjusted by the released cell material, does the growth of the culture begin once more. *Kellner* also worked through the experiment physico-chemically, and saw that in this regard the constitution of the culture medium is the determinant factor for the way the cells react; when the deviations are too large, cytolysis begins.

Leukolysis, which can be placed in parallel to cytolysis in serum and cultures, thus appears to be dependent on physico-chemical factors such as, pH, rH, and surface and border surface activity.

This is confirmed by the fact that its suppression with simultaneous lymphocyte regression causes the death of the animal, as *an elementary process of the organism*. It is obviously initiated by a milieu change in the blood, based on physicochemical or energy factors. In this sense – formulated in a general way – one can speak of a regulatory cell-milieu reaction, to which we had already given attention earlier for the basic (connective) tissue. Here, as there, the milieu (here the blood plasma) must be brought back to an adequate state through the substances of the destroyed – not degenerating – cells. It should not be overlooked that this is not a matter of small quantities of material released by cell breakdown. *Kellner* (pesonal information) estimated that up to *half a gram of* leukocyte (moist) weight was disintegrating at the moment of counting, with their substances taking effect.

A series of further questions emerge, e.g., as already said: how many leukocytes actually disintegrate? Is the quantity parallel with the number of lysis forms, or are these amounts reversely proportioned? Namely: do the lysis forms decrease because the disintegration takes place more rapidly, or do the leukocytes become more resistant? From *Koch* we know that the number of breakdown cells is parallel to the serum peroxidase content, which comes from the granulocytes. Thus, according to *Koch,* the number of breakdown cells could be used as an indicator for intravital leukocyte destruction. A further question concerns the fate and the function of the *nucleic acids* that are constantly released in lysis; their quantity is certainly not small. A third question also has to be considered, namely, what is the source of the monocyte-stimulating *substances;* as is seen, this should be given an importance equal to that of leukolysing factors. Finally, the cytolytic processes in leukocytes in blood diseases can not be ignored; here, the breakdown forms are particularly abundant. The questions have to be the object of special hematological work".

However, the leukocytolysis as such is not significant, but its contribution to ground regulation is significant. This presupposes the readiness ("sensitivity") of a certain percentage of leukocytes, corresponding to the initial individual state, for physiological lysis. Consideration of this "pool" allows an estimation of the reactivity of the extracellular matrix.

A test of this sort, which is based on the binding of a lectin-polysaccharide complex on the surface of the blood cell, permits the recording of lysis-ready leukocytes in the differential blood picture (*Heine* 1988).

Regulation of Tumor Extracellular Matrix

The fibroblast is the regulation center of the normal extracellular matrix. In contrast to this, in fast-growing, malignant tumors, every cell is able to synthesize tumor-specific extracellular matrix by shedding "tumor matrix vesicles" (Fig. 5, *Heine* 1987a, 1988a). This high-energy reaction situation is superior to normal ground regulation. Through para- and autostimulation, the tumor process can spread peripherally with progressive inclusion of adjacent tissue Fig. 5A, 5B). The normal extracellular matrix is destroyed by proteolytic and hydrolytic enzymes from the disintegrated tumor matrix vesicles. Here, plasmin is important, it can break down proteoglycans through release of plasminogen activators from the tumor matrix vesicles (*Heine* 1987a). Correspondingly, in malignancies, an "isolation" of the extracellular matrix to polysaccharide complexes can be observed. With increasing de-differentiation and malignancy, this leads to a predominance of hyaluronic acid (a highly negatively-charged, elongated glucosoaminoglycan with no protein binding) (*Heine* 1987a). Here it is worth keeping in mind that hyaluronic acid is a phylogenetically ancient part of the extracellular matrix of all multicellular organisms. In human beings it appears at the end of the second week of development, with the formation of the mesenchyme (Fig. 4). Proteoglycans are only formed later. The importance of this polyanion lies in the fact that it has a mitogenic effect, and is at the same time an inhibitor of differentiation (*Toole* 1983, *Heine* 1987a). In malignancies this phenomenon reappears at the wrong site and at the wrong time (*Heine* 1987a). Since, apart from the importance of radiological and surgical reduction of the size of the tumor mass, i.v. cytostatics also damage intact extracellular matrix, adjuvant activation of the ground regulation of healthy tissue, with stimulation of increased extracellular matrix regulation must be recommended before, with and after school-medicine treatment. All the so-called natural therapies are suitable for this, since they stimulate the self-healing capacities and reserves of the organism. Even in sick people, such normal potencials and reserves are usually available, and can be therapeutically stimulated (cf. *Leupold* 1945, 1954).

Significance of Chronobiology

It should not be underestimated how important social contacts, mental, dietetic and climatic factors are for maintenance and activation of ground regulation, as well as an individual life rhythm. This points to a close connection between endogenous and exogenous rhythms. Since open-energy systems are compelled to oscillation due to their instability, corresponding to the principle of activation and inhibition, the rhythms at the molecular level are subject to superior rhythms, such as day and night rhythm or seasonal rhythms. The most important intracellular pacer is the rhythmic synthesis of ATP by the cell mitochondria (*Priebe* 1980); bound to the cell membrane, it is the circadian rhythm of "second messengers" as it is the situation with the sympathetic-associated cyclic adenosine monophosphate (cAMP) (*Lemmer* 1983). In the extracellular space it is in the end the rhythm in the relationship of sugar bipolymers to the molecule swarms of fluid-crystal water and ions. For example, this relationship can be seen in the control of the circadian rhythm over urine excretion. In 1983, *Quincke* had already observed an inverse rhythm of urine excretion in patients. Nocturnal polyuria is still an important symptom in patients with heart failure.

Circadian temperature variations are also an important indicator of molecular rhythmus in the relationship between the extracellular matrix and the cells. This is made clearer by investigations carried out by *Gautherie* and *Gros* (1977) in breast cancer. In 26 women, after a precise grading and staging of the tumor, as well as synchronization as regards activity, sleeping time, meal times and room temperature, the skin temperatures of the diseased and the non-diseased breasts were measured continuously by telemetry for nine days. In 11 patients with a slow-growing, well-differentiated carcinoma, analysis of the findings also showed a circadian rhythm in the temperature on the affected side, but the amplitude was reduced and the temperature maximum appeared earlier. In 15 patients with rapidly-growing tumors with histologically undifferentiated cells, no circadian rhythm was observed in the skin temperature on the affected side.

This agrees with the "de-differentiation" of the extracellular matrix with predominance of hyaluronic acid. In developmental history, hyaluronic acid predominates initially in the extracellular matrix, so rhythms are also subject to a maturing process. An example of this is the circadian rhythm in body temperature that can be observed in adults, which is only reached after the 7th year of life with regard to amplitude and phase (*Abe* et al. 1978). Anthroposophic medicine has demonstrated convincing findings for a 7 year rhythm in mental and spiritual development in connection with the body (*Fintelmann* 1988). A conscious control of the relationship between the extracellular matrix and the cell is made possible by the pain sensation, which is also subject to a circadian rhythm. Unclear disturbances of health, endogenous depression and diffuse pains of psychogenic type point to disturbances of the molecular rhythm in the relationship between the cell and the extracellular matrix. Among other areas, they appear in disturbances of the sleep-wake rhythm (Overviews in *Lemmer* 1983 and *Hildebrandt* 1987).

Topography of Extracellular Matrix Distribution

Loose "soft" connective tissue, which still corresponds to the embryonic mesenchyme, is particularly rich in extracellular matrix, and is thus particularly reactive. It has a typical distribution pattern: it accompanies all capillaries, forms the reticular cell tissue underlying epithelial cell groups like the epidermis and mucosa (e.g. the tunica propria of the esophagus and gastrointestinal canal), the splenic pulp, lymphatic tissue, fat tissue, the uterine mucosa, the ovarian cortex, the tooth pulp and the *Virchow-Robin* spaces in the CNS. As the loose endoneurium, endomysium and peritendineum internum it accompanies the vessels between nerve, muscle and tendon fibers. It forms interstitial connective tissue, which, among other functions, subdivides glandular tissue into lobules as vascular- and nerve-conducting interstitial connective tissue. The adventitia of the larger vessels, the serous membrane tissues, the endocardium, the soft brain membranes, the interstitial tissues of the lung periphery, the joint capsule synovial membranes and the innermost layer of the periosteum consist of loose connective tissue.

The finely-structured connective tissue of the organ capsules forms a transition to stiff and hard connective tissue types. Tendons, fascia, ligaments, aponeuroses, dura mater, the stratum texticulare of the skin, the cornea, cartilage, bone and dentin already have the character of organs. These organs are also provided with loose connective tissue accompanying vessels and nerves (e.g. *Haver's* and *Volkmann's* channel in bone, dentin canaliculi in the teeth). Only the cornea and postnatal joint cartilages are free of blood vessels.

The conncection between hard substance penetrated by soft connective tissue accompanied by vessels and nerves is a clear illustration of the importance of the loose connective tissue bearing extracellular matrix. Its purpose includes maintaining the functional capacity of the hard substance; here, this is obvious. Recently, the closely circumscribed perforations in the superficial body fascia (diameter 3–7 mm) have been shown to be particularly significant, as only there, invested in loose connective tissue, can the vessel-nerve bundles of the skin penetrate deeply. They present the morphological correlation of acupuncture points (*Heine* 1988b). After connection with the vessels and nerves, the latter finally reach the spinal nerves of the CNS. Analogously, fine vascular nervous bundles, invested in loose connective tissue, leave the area of the ossified sulci of the dura mater through the bone and appear in the skin of the scalp. The exit points in the bone also correspond to acupuncture (*Heine* 1988b).

Since these "points" (or rather, perforations) are always found in the same place, irrespective of racial differences, they seem to have a genetic origin.

Obviously, the acupuncture points can also become diseased themselves (perhaps there is a causative explanation here for peripheral neuropathies, Sudeck's atrophy-dystrophy syndrome, painful trigger-points, etc.). These findings also offer a rational basis for neurotherapy and related methods (see contribution from *Bergsmann*).

Structural Components of the Extracellular Matrix

Glycosaminoglycans (GAGs)

GAGs present unbranched, negatively-charged, linear carbohydrate chains with characteristic, repeated disaccharide units of hexosamines (D-glucosamine, D-galactosamine) and uronic acids (D-glucuronic acid, L-iduronic acid). The most important GAGs for the extracellular matrix are: hyaluronic acid, chondroitin sulphate, dermatan sulphate, keratan sulphate and heparin. Hyaluronic acid is the largest and most important GAG, with a molecular weight of about 100,000 to several million Daltons, and consists of disaccharide polymers of N-acetylglucosamine and D-glucouronic acid. Only hyaluronic acid and heparin appear as free, non-protein-bound GAG, and are correspondingly water-soluble. Keratan sulphate is an exception, since the uronic acid is replaced there by galactose. Heparan sulphate and heparin contain N-sulphated groups in the glucosamine remnants (*Matthews* 1975, *Hascall* and *Hascall* 1983).

Sulfate and carboxyl groups give the GAGs a strongly negative charge. Through mutual charge loss, the polymers are stretched, which determines their biological characteristics and reciprocal effects with other molecules. Hyaluronic acid is the phylogenetically oldest carbohydrate biopolymer of multicellular life forms, and can be demonstrated in the basic substance of sponges (*Matthews* 1975). Hyaluronic acid has an outstanding binding capacity for proteoglycans. This presents the phylogenetic and evolutionary start-point for the higher development of multicellular organisms (*Matthews* 1975).

From the developmental historical point of view, hyaluronic acid is thus the first extracellular matrix component to appear in the embryonic development of vertebrates. Its significance lies in the regulation of cell division and cell movement, as well as inhibition of premature cell specialization (its significance in tumor events has already been pointed out). Due to its higher negative charge, hyaluronic acid is particularly capable of water binding and ion exchange. Compared to other biopolymers, hyaluronic acid in aqueous solution covers a very large domain (unfolding scope). The water requirement for full extension is so large that the individual molecule already assumes a zig-zag form with a concentration of 0.1% (W/N), and starts to overlap.

These domains of the GAGs and proteoglycans have an exclusion character against molecules of a certain size. They thus form a primitive first defence system. The domains are elastically deformable, and thus offer a shock-absorbing, viscoelastic system with an energy-absorbing effect. With proteoglycans, hyaluronic acid forms an important lubricant, and, among other effects is an important part of the synovia. The common denominator of the highly etiologically-variable diseases of the rheumatic type thus lies in pathological changes in the hyaluronic acid and the proteoglycans bound to it (*Heine* and *Schaeg* 1979, review in *Hascall* and *Hascall* 1983).

Heparin is a GAG of special physiological importance. As the only biopolymeric sugar, it is stored in a specific cell type of the mast cells or the basophilic granulocytes in the form of membrane-enclosed vesicles, and released when needed. In the author's opinion, the mast cell can also be a basophilic granulocyte that has wandered out of the bloodstream, whose formation site is the bone marrow, or can also be formed locally from primitive mesenchymal cells, or correspond to the reticular cells of the bone marrow. From personal observations, fibrocytes and local macrophages (histiocytes) have the capacity to take up mast cell granules, as well as heparin that has been injected transepidermally or subcutaneously (*Heine* 1984, 1986).

Mast cells are capable of ameboid movement and are neurotropic, i.e. they travel to the termini of autonomic axons. Since these are found more commonly in the immediate vicinity of capillaries and in the adventitia of larger vessels, mast cells are mainly found in the immediate vicinity of capillaries and large vessels. Catecholamines produce a significant stimulus for degranulation, and these are released in the extracellular matrix, e.g., under conditions of increased stress. However, pH changes to acid, the binding of certain antigenic substances ("allergens") via the IgE receptors of the mast cell surface, inflammation mediators (e.g. certain leukotrienes as "slow reacting substance of anaphylaxis"), and many other factors, lead to mast cell degranulation (*Heine* and *Schaeg* 1979, *König* 1983). Thereby, the coagulation-inhibiting function of heparin is wrongly placed in the foreground. Heparin takes part in all the regulations processes in the extracellular matrix. Heparin has a regulatory influence in the lipolysis of circulating lipoproteins through activation of lipoprotein lipase in the endothelium; it promotes the aggregation of lymphocytes and activates muscle cell protein kinases. Heparin promotes the synthesis of extracellular matrix by fibrocytes, takes part in the activation of about 50 enzymes, and intervenes in the translation and transcription mechanisms of DNA and RNA. Heparin promotes the breakdown of the anaphylactic complement factor C3, inhibits the effects of interferon, regulated thrombospondin synthesis in endothelia and smooth muscle cells, and intervenes in collagen synthesis and collagen fiber polymerization. In addition, it is well documented that heparin modulates circulating growth factors, has a significant role in the control of plasminogen activators, and is involved in bindings with angiogenesis factors, histidine-rich glycoproteins, fibronectin and platelet factor 4 (Overview in *Engelbrecht* 1977).

Sugars of the Cell Surface – the Glycocalyx

The cell sugar surface film mediates functionally between the cell interior and the extracellular space (Fig. 1). It provides the cell-specific and organ-specific receptor coating of the cell, and this has a significant influence on its function and integrity. The glycocalyx sugars consist of branched oligosaccharides with terminal N-acetylneuraminic acid, and branch into the proteins and lipids (glycoproteins and -lipids) of the cell membrane. Individual glycocalyx components have been known for a considerable time as blood group substances and transplant antigens. Loss of the terminal neuraminic acid is an indication, for example, of the ageing of a cell, and this is recognized by the RES cells, leading to elimination. Analogously, there are filamented glycoproteins on the inside of the cell membrane, related to spectrin, vinculin and actomyosin. They bind to both the integral proteins of the cell membrane and to the filaments of the cytoskeleton. In this way, important membrane functions are controlled significantly, such as its fluidity and thus its capacity for depolarization and repolarization, the activation of secondary messengers in the membrane, receptor properties, and many other factors (Overview in *Hay* 1983). Due to its negative charge, the glycocalyx has its own electrical potential, which differs from that of the extracellular matrix and the cell membrane , which reacts with its own change in potential after a certain charge alteration in the extracellular matrix. This suffices to activate the system of membrane secondary messengers in all connective tissue, defence and epithelial cells (particularly adenylate cyclase - cAMP and -cGMP system, inosite phosphate, G proteins). The membranes of nerve cells and their processes, the membranes of cardiac muscle cells, smooth muscle cells and striated muscle fibers, on the other hand, are depolarized. This is followed by a cell-specific response (e.g. adjusted synthesis of extracellular matrix, muscle contraction, the production of a nerve potential).

The glycocalyx has binding sites for GAGs (particularly hyaluronic acid, heparan sulfate and chondroitin sulfate); at the time, the GAGs are bound covalently to hydroxyaminic acid remnants of the membrane glycoproteins.

The glycocalyx GAGs are coupled to one another by bivalent cations (mainly calcium ions). The glycocalyx GAGs participate in growth control, mitosis frequency and the active movements of cells. The cell surface GAGs also bind to proteoglycans and structural glycoproteins of the extracellular matrix. In this way, contact is made between the extracellular matrix in the extracellular space and the cytoskeleton inside the cell via the membrane glycoproteins and membrane lipids. There are indications that proteoglycans and certain network proteins of the extracellular matrix (e.g. fibronectin) can penetrate the cell membrane directly, and thus make immediate contact with the filamentous cytoskeleton (*Yamada* 1983, *Iozzo* 1985). In this way, an exceptionally precise and rapid extracellular-intracellular, or vice versa, information transfer would be possible (similar to light conduction along fiberglass fibers) (*Heine* 1986). In tumor cells these relationships are disturbed significantly since the product of a certain oncogen (rasoncogen) masks the vinculin at the inner side of the cell membrane in such a way that the cytoskeleton can no longer adhere regularly to the membrane, and there is thus a severe alteration in all cell functions (*Osborn* and *Weber* 1986). Among other effects, this favors tumor matrix vesicle formation (*Heine* 1987).

Disturbances of the extracellular matrix can also lead to such alterations of the glycocalxy sugars that there are major changes in cell behaviour, among other effects. After loss of the terminal sialic acid, sugar components can be released that can be recognized from the construction of the carbohydrate chains, e.g. by bacteria, and can bind to these; but plant, microbial and host lectins can also bind to the glycocalyx sugars, and provoke a wide variety of cell reactions (division and synthesis capacity). Under lectins, one understands glycoconjugates and proteins that mainly have the function of recognizing sugar structures on the cell surface or in soluble glycoconjugates. Here, there is no relationship to the specific recognition mechanism of the immune system; they have no enzymatic activity. Obviously, they play a major role in so-called immune modulation (*Uhlenbruck* et al. 1986, *Heine* 1988). More important is the fact that lectins of the tumor cell glycocalyx of this type can be responsible for organotropic metastasis spread. For instance, in the glycocalyx of the liver cells there is a sugar component as a lectin that forms a receptor for serum asialoglycoprotein, and also has mitogenic capacities. It is assumed that certain lectins "are decisive for both the adhesion of circulating tumor cells, and, with appropriate stimulation, for the growth behaviour, as they have a reciprocal effect

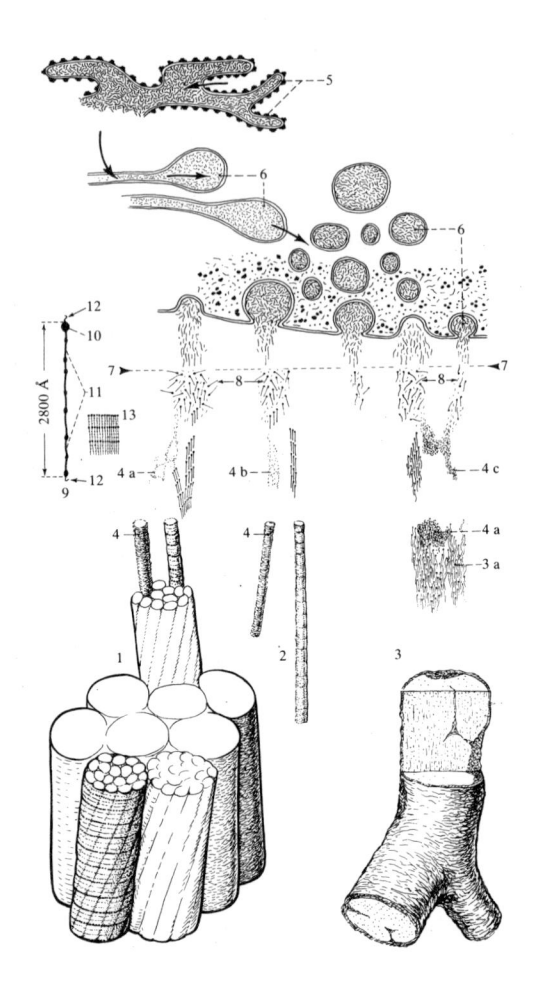

Fig. 6: Diagram of formation of: 1 collagen, 2 reticular, 3 elastic fibers, and 4 proteoglycans. In the rough endoplasmic reticulum (5), tropocollagen (tropoelastin) and proteoglycans are synthesized through amino acids being taken-up into the fibroblast cytoplasm, completed in the smooth ER and extruded via the vesicles of the Golgi apparatus. The various types of fibers are orientated and formed in the close vicinity of the cells (7), and this seems to depend on local conditions. This gives the proteoglycans (4 a, b, c) great quantitative and qualitative significance. 8 Tropocollagen molecules; 9 greatly enlarged tropocollagen molecule; head (10) and tail (11) with telopeptides (12). Fibril formation with collagenous and reticular fibers through joining of tropocollagen molecules with individual displacements of a quarter of their length. 13 long-spacing collagen is formed by lateral aggregation of tropocollagen molecules without stepped displacement. Elastin-specific formation of desmosin and isodesmosin takes place in the formation of elastic fibers (3) through intermeshing of 3a and 4a.

with the exposed carbohydrate structures of the tumor cells" (*Uhlenbruck* et al. 1986). On the other hand, tumor cells can protect themselves from recognition by lymphocytes with a hyaluronic acid screen (*McBride* and *Bard* 1979).

Basement Membranes

Basement membranes are a special form of extracellular matrix (Fig. 6). They are formed as a co-product of epithelial cells and underlying connective tissue. An underlying basement membrane is urgently necessary for the normal growth of epithelia (*Toole* 1983). Basement membranes also cover certain types of cells: Schwann cells, terminal "naked" axons, striated muscle fibers, cardiac muscle cells and smooth muscle cells. Since it is a matter here of cell forms whose cell membranes depolarize after appropriate stimuli (opening of Na^+-, K^+- and Ca^{2+}- channels), the basement membrane with its sugar polymers may represent an important mobile calcium reservoir.

The basement membrane underlying vascular endothelium has special importance as a molecular sieve. It can merge with epithelial basement membranes. There are common basement sections between alveolar epithelium and alveolar capillaries, in the renal glomeruli between the internal leaf of Bowman's capsule (podocytes) and the glomerular capillaries, and as the blood-brain barrier between the capillaries of the CNS and astrocyte processes closed together with the perivascular glial lamina. Every alteration of these basement membrane sections results in severe organ damage (e.g. shock lung, renal autoimmune disease, oxygen and glucose deficiency in the brain).

Heine (1987b) was able to show findings on why the appearance of inflammation is not transferred from connective tissue to epithelium. Using the example of the basement membrane of the epidermis and the renal glomeruli it could be shown that their greater vitamin C (ascorbic acid) content is apparently suitable for snaring the radical ions of an inflammatory process. In the same paper it was shown that in mammary carcinoma, the tumor cells loose their vitamin C to the epidermal basement membrane as they approach it.

Proteoglycans (PGs)

In all organisms, the water-sugar-polymer system experiences energy stabilisation through binding to a protein backbone which is bound to hyaluronic acid via binding proteins (Figs. 2, 3). These proteoglycan biopolymers also acquire an increased electronegative charge through sulfation and amination as well as a terminal supply of acetyl neuraminic acid (sialic acid) (reviewed by *Heine* and *Schaeg* 1979).

The molecular construction is important for understanding the functional relationships between water molecules and proteoglycan molecules (Fig. 3). Proteoglycans have a brush-like structure, with the approximately 300 nm long protein backbone as the "handle" of the brush; due to their mutually electronegative repulsion, the olygosaccharide chains form the stretched, approximately 60 nm to 100 nm long "bristles". The molecular weight of proteoglycans lies between 10^6 and 10^9 Daltons (*Hascall* and *Hascall* 1983). This molecular form is obviously particularly suitable for binding water, and through this, a single PG molecule can take up a very large amount of space ("domain") compared to its molecular weight. The "domain" has a significant role in determining the "molecular sieve character", as well as the viscoelastic, shock-absorbing and energy-absorbing behaviour of the extracellular matrix (reviews in *Balasz* 1970, *Heine* and *Schaeg* 1979, *Hay* 1983).

The molecular form of tissue water has been investigated in detail by *Trincher* (1978). The special suitability of networks of water molecules for information conduction and storage between cells is, according to *Trincher* (1978), due to their molecular structure, which consists of up to about 50% fluid crystals at body temperature. To maintain water in this condition, it should have its lowest energy requirement at 37.5°C (*Trincher* 1978). False information stored in the liquid crystals could therefore be cancelled by temperature increase and thus by transfer to more homogeneous fluid (*Trincher* 1978). The cell biophoton emission namend by *Popp* (1976) could also play a part in distant informative reciprocal effects via these liquid-crystalline intercellular "bridges".

The mark of crystalline liquids is the formation of parallel swarms of molecules, arranged in two dimensions, which are limited to small areas and are not stable in time. They are in a state of constant formation and dissolution, and show statistically disordered positions relative to one another. The size of these swarms lies in approximately the light-wave field. Even weak external powers are sufficient to bring about a greater state of order (*Hollemann-Richter* 1963).

Histological tissue freeze-drying shows that tissue water is in a special state. In tissue drying, the formation of ice crystals can only be voided in the water, after rapid cooling of the tissue in liquid air (-150°C). The drying process that follows has to be carried out under negative pressure below the temperature of the eutectic point of the tissue water.

In this process, the tissue water changes directly to a vaporized state, and can be pumped off. If the drying process is broken off too soon, there is an increase in temperature and gradual breaking of the vacuum in the area of the eutectic point of the tissue water (approximately between -58°C and -52°C, there is a short-lasting breakdown of the vacuum with the formation of ice crystals and destruction of cell structures) (*Heine* 1974). The low eutectic point of tissue water does not only depend on its composition, since media with similar composition, as, e.g., used in cell cultures, already start to freeze at about -8°C (personal observation). The remarkable eutectic behaviour of tissue water thus appears to depend on the arrangement of liquid crystalline water between the sugar polymers of the proteoglycan brushes.

The basis of all intercellular near and long-distance reciprocal effects in a multicellular organism is obviously a characteristic of the water-sugar-biopolymers of the extracellular matrix, which are capable of information conduction and storage due to their chemical structure. The system is an open-energy one, and capable of removal of the energy released in all metabolic processes by radical reactions. From a certain size, the energy fluctuations that appear in this process can spread rapidly through the extracellular matrix through changes in the state of the liquid crystalline water, and can be used by the cell as information.

Minimal amounts of energy are sufficient for this, as shown by *Pischinger's* puncture phenomenon (1983) and *Huneke's* second phenomenon of neural therapy (1983). The energy displacements iniated in this way do not need to be demonstrable biologically, but they can be measurable as biophysical fluctuations of the redox potential of the connective tissue, among other methods. It is therefore logical that particularly in chronic diseases and tumors, which are obviously always accompanied by alterations in the PG/GAGpattern (*Heine* 1987), there is an altered redox potential in the extracellular matrix, which frequently can not be regulated (*Pischinger* 1983, *Perger* 1983).

The extracellular matrix therefore presents a labile arrangement system with sugar-biopolymers, water and the substances dissolved in it as the main components. Here, system means "capacity", "standing in relationship" or "having a relationship to one another" (*Gutmann* and *Resch* 1988).

Here, the system organisation between water and the substances dissolved in it, namely molecules (or ions) of dissolved solid bodies, liquids and dissolved gases, is of special importance. In aqueous solution, hydrophilic substances such as dissolved ions and generally hydrated molecules, e.g. sugar, urea, silicic acid, etc., can be termed "structure breakers" (*Gutmann* and *Resch* 1988). The sugar biopolymers of the extracellular matrix certainly condense the molecular swarms of water in their surroundings to individual molecular "domains" (Fig. 3), whose arrangement is, however, signfiicantly more noticeable as regards these changes than it would be in the sugar-water system in pure water.

In reverse, gases dissolved in water, e.g. O_2, N_2, CO_2, or other hydrophobic substances, can be termed "structure makers" as regards stored water (*Gutmann* and *Resch* 1988). These authors point out that "structure makers" bring about a certain sort of ordered dynamism of water structure. Radiological spectra of crystallised gaseous hydrates show that gas molecules are embedded in hollow spaces which are larger than would be necessary for their accommodation. Through this, gas molecules have a certain freedom of movement. For example, on the inner surfaces of the spaces, the distance between oxygen molecules is less; this leads to internal surface tensions which make maintenance of the space possible. *Gutmann* and *Resch* (1988) also point out that the limited rotary oscillation of gas molecules in the spaces can be tuned to certain oscillation patterns, and has to attune rhythmically to the oscillation behaviour of the fluid. This, again, depends on the binding behaviour of the "structure breakers", e.g. the sugar biopolymers of the extracellular matrix. Basically, due to the alterations brought about by the alternating relationship between "structure breakers" and "structure makers", the entire extracellular matrix and cell system is affected, even if in different regional ways. "Structure breakers" and "structure makers" thus exercise varying, mutually complementary "functions" in the sense of retention of homeostasis. "These structure breakers have greater hierarchical importance as regards structural character, and structure makers as regards structural information" *(Gutmann* and *Resch* 1988).

Proteoglycan Synthesis

Synthesis of the protein and polysaccharide parts takes place simultaneously at the membranes of the fibroblast endoplasmic reticulum (Fig. 6) (review in *Hascall* and *Hascall* 1983). Synthesis of the protein backbone of PG corresponds to the simpler proteins and is bound to various RNA-type messengers. First of all, a precursor of the protein backbone is formed at the ribosome and given up to the raw endoplasmic reticulum (Fig. 6). While the protein backbone is elongated, the attachment of oligosaccharide chains via N and O bindings begins, through the action of glycosyltransferases in the membranes, with transfer to the smooth parts of the cisterns. Gonadotrophic hormones obviously play a role here. The entire synthesis process can be inhibited by tunicamycin (*Takatsuki* and *Tamura* 1977).

While mannose-rich oligosaccharides start their chain growth at asparagine remnants of the protein backbone with a nitrogen-glycosylamine binding, keratan sulfate chains are bound to serine (or threonine) through glycosidic-binding of N-acetyl-galactosamine. In the former, dolichol pyrophosphate intermediates are the initiating, energy-rich bindings; in the latter the initial binding energy comes from uridine diphosphate (UDP), bound to N-acetyl-galactosamine. The reaction is started by the transfer of xylose to serine of the protein backbone by a glycosidic binding. 6 different glycosyl transferases take part in the further chain construction of the carbohydrate part. In this, energy-rich monosaccharides (UDP) are attached to the non-reduced ends of the chains. Adenosine-3-phosphate-5-phosphate sulfate (PAPS) forms the biological sulfate carrier at the same time. The sulfotransferase activity also takes place in the membrane tubes of the smooth endoplasmic reticulum. Finally, the PGs are packed into vesicles of the Golgi apparatus and ejected with tropocollagen and tropoelastin. After the oligosaccharide chain starts, PGs can be released from the cell into the extracellular space in 1–2 minutes (*Dorfmann* 1983, *Iozzo* 1985). Using radioactively-marked proline on rat fibroblasts, *Hauss* et al. (1968) were able to show a new synthesis of collagen after noise stress within minutes.

With radioactively marked sulfate as precursor in an experimental stress model, *Heine* and *Henrich* (1980) showed that extracellular matrix, synthesized from myocytes from the media of the rat femoral artery shows a significant increase in sulfated extracellular matrix components (chondroitin sulfate and dermatan sulfate proteins) after one hour of sympathetic stimulation. Vascular wall myocytes, as fibrocyte descendants, are also capable of extracellular matrix synthesis. In particular, dermatan sulfate is suitable for trapping lipids and calcium ions, which encourages arteriosclerotic changes.

Ground substance synthesis caused by stress must lead to functional disturbances in the extracellular matrix in continuing stress, and thus cause changes in its molecular sieve character. Finally, the process enters a vicious circle, laying the basis for chronic diseases and tumor development. After experimental multiple trauma in dogs, and in lung biopsies of severely traumatised accident victims, *Heine* et al. (1980) showed that there is an increase in collagen in the alveolar septa within 30 minutes, and from this the clinical picture of shock lung can develop weeks later.

The structural properties of PGs can be seen in the example of a monomer chondroitin sulfate proteoglycan molecule (Ch-PG), and 4 regions can be differentiated in the protein backbone (Iozzo 1986):

a) A binding region for hyaluronic acid. It consists of two binding proteins (a smaller one with a molecular weight of 42,000 D and a larger one with 50,000 D; *Baker* and *Caterson* 1979). These "left proteins" do not carry sugar side-chains.

b) The region of the N terminal is attached to this, with 10 to 15 N-glycoside-bound oligosaccharide chains.

c) Distally, follows the keratan sulfate binding region. It occupies about 10% of the protein backbone.

d) After this follows the chondroitin sulfate binding region, which stretches over about 60% of the protein backbone.

In spite of its relative size, the mass of the protein backbone is only 5–10% of the mass of a PG monomer. About 100 chondroitin sulfate chains and 50 to 60 keratan sulfate chains have O-glycosidic bindings to the protein backbone of a monomer. There are a further 50 to 60 O-bound oligosaccharides of the "mucin type" distributed over the protein backbone, i.e. they carry terminal sialic acid remnants.

In human articular cartilage and the nasal cartilage of cattle, the chondroitin sulfate binding region contains bound covalent phosphate remnants; about 1 phosphate chain to 20 oligosaccharide chains. The C2 atom of xylose thus appears to be the preferred site for phosphorylation. In chondrosarcoma of the rat, about 80% of the chondroitin sulfate chains are phosphorylated (overview in *Iozzo* 1985).

A Ch-PG molecule with a length of about 300 nm has a molecular weight of about 250,000 D. The oligosaccharide side chains are stretched and 50 to 60 nm in length. A single chain has a molecular weight of about 20,000 D. The spacing of the oligosaccharide chain is about 30 nm, obvisously due to loading. Overall, the molecular weight of a monomer PG molecule is about 2.5×10^6 (*Hascall* and *Hascall* 1983). Via their binding proteins, monomer PGs bind very specifically to a long (up to 1mm) hyaluronic acid band (Fig. 3). Here, intervals of about 30 nm spacing are maintained, which correspond to a disaccharide unit of hyaluronic acid; each repeats itself after five more disaccharide units. The dissociation constant is 10^{-6} to 10^{-7}, and is thus extremely stable (*Christner* et al. 1979). Up to now, no anionic biopolymer is known that would compete with these bindings. An aggregate of PG and hyaluronic acid contains about 40 PG monomers and has a molecular weight of approximately 10^8 D (*Hascall* and *Hascall* 1983). The half-life of hyaluronic acid is 6–12 days, of chondroitin sulfate 7–17 days, and of keratan sulfate protein 60–120 days. Growth hormones and estrogens elongate chondroitin sulfate protein chains and shorten keratan sulfate protein chains (*Iozzo* 1985).

Functional Aspects of Ch-PG-Hyaluronic Acid Complexes

As described, Ch-PGs with hyaluronic acid form large supermolecular complexes, up to 0,1 μm long. In relation to their molecular weight they occupy an enormous hydrodynamic volume (domain) (Fig. 3). If the tissue water is reduced in amount, there is a strong intermolecular interaction between the stiff, polyanionic oligosaccharide chains. When water is added they re-expand accordingly.

Since the PGs and hyaluronic acid give the extracellular matrix a net-like supermolecular superstructure, cover cell surfaces, form the intercellular substance, and invest and interlace through collagen and elastin fibers, this "buffering" viscoelastic property of the PGs and hyaluronic acid is extremely important for normal tissue and cell function. This is particularly useful in the functions of articular cartilage and cardiac and vascular pulsation. The local concentrations of PGs and hyaluronic acid in a tissue area therefore determine its mechanical dynamics. One must always bear in mind that the individual synthesis and metabolic stages of PGs, their protein backbone, their oligosaccharide side-chains, their binding to hyaluronic acid, the free GAGs, as well as structural and network proteins (collagen, elastin, fibronectin, etc.) can be disturbed or altered by endogenous errors (collections of genetic errors or mistakes in the cellular control mechanisms due to ageing or genetic processes), exogenous factors (environmental contamination, especially by chemical radicals, false nutrition, stress, viral and bacterial infections, radiation, alkylising substances, etc.), which can cause a tremendous number and variety of connective tissue, vascular, cartilage and bone diseases. The biological flow balance of PGs is mainly determined by proteolytic enzymes, particularly the serine proteases such as plasmin, since most of the oligosaccharide chains attach themselves to the protein backbone of a PG via serine. The GAGs and the oligosaccharide chains are split by hydrolytic enzymes. The largest spectrum of these enzymes is found in the lysosomes of neutrophil granulocytes and macrophages. This casts a special light on physiological leukocytolysis as an important regulator in the formation and breakdown of the extracellular matrix.

Dermatan Sulfate – Proteoglycan

In contrast to Ch-PG, dermatan sulfate – proteoglycan (Dm-PG) is not bound to hyaluronic acid. The protein backbone is very long, with a molecular weight of equal to or more than 300.000 D. In contrast to Ch-PG it has about 10 to 20 oligosaccharide side-chains, which all contain iduronic acid. The molecular weight of the side-chains is more than double that of the Ch-PG side chains (about 56.000 D). The neuraminic acid content is also higher. 300 to 400 oligosaccharide side chains of the mucin type have O-glycosidic bindings to the serine and threonine of the protein backbone, and about 50 side-chains have N-glycosidic bindings. Dm-PG thus shows great similarity to the mucus produced by the glandular epithelia ("mucins") (overview in *Iozzo*, 1985).

Functional Aspects of Dermatan Sulfate – Proteoglycan

In contrast to the more densely packed Ch-PG, Dm-PG has an open structure with the development of even larger domains. Dm-PG appears in larger amounts in the extracellular matrix of the connective tissue of the skin, the cornea, the sclera, tendons, cartilage and bones. Dm-PG has a special function in follicle ripening and ovulation. It collects increasingly in the fluid of the cavities in the tertiary follicle (*Graafian* follicle), keeps these under tension, and gives the follicle liquid the necessary viscosity for ovulation. If the follicle liquid increases in quantity under the influence of gonadotrophic hormones, the follicle epithelial cells synthesize more Dm-PG (*Iozzo* 1985).

Dm-PG plays a significant role in the maturing of collagen fibrils. It binds in the area of the d-band (gap region of the collagen fibril) and through this couples the fibrils to one another in higher fiber arrangements (*Öbrink* 1975).

Heparan Sulfate – Proteoglycan

Heparan sulfate – proteoglycan molecules (Hp-PG), similarly to heparan sulfate as GAG, have a special affinity for cell surfaces. Precise structural investigations were carried out on HP-PG of human colon carcinoma cells (*Iozzo* 1985). The protein backbone has a molecular weight of about 240.000 D. Apart from about 100 to 200 oligosaccharide chains with O-glycosidic bindings to the protein backbone, which contain glucosamine, galactosamine and sialinic acid, there are 10 to 15 pure heparan sulfate chains. In contrast to all other PG types, the protein backbone of Hp-PG contains a hydrophobe domain which anchors the HP-PG in the cell membrane. The binding is very strong and can only be dissolved by proteolysis. This anchoring site possibly extends into the cell cytoplasm, with a reciprocal effect with the filaments of the cytoskeleton (*Iozzo* 1985).

Functional Aspects

Hp-PG also has other binding capacities, apart from this transmembranous aspect the heparan sulfate side-chains of PG can bind to "receptors" in the glycocalyx through ion formation, and can be freed from these bindings by addition of polyanions, such as heparin. In vitro, 6×10^7 binding sites per cm^2 were established for heparin (*Psuya* et al. 1987). Heparan sulfate chains of a variety of monomers can make bindings with one another. Since all PG types have one or more heparan sulfate side chains, Hp-PG and heparan sulfate have an important function in the maintenance of cell groups and their anchoring to basement membranes or their structural parts (collagen, fibronectin, laminin). Due to these "surface associated" properties of Hp-PG and heparan sulfate, it is assumed that these polymers have a direct influence on cell growth and multiplication (*Chiarugi* et al. 1976, *Iozzo* 1985).

Keratan sulfate – Proteoglycan

The special structural property of keratan sulfate – proteoglycan (Kt-PG) is that its oligosaccharide side-chains contain D-galactose, and that none of the side-chains are bound to the aminoacid serine of the protein backbone via xylose. Rather more, there are O-glycosidic bindings between N-acetylgalactosamine and the hydroxyl groups of serine or threonine. In the cornea, there are N-glycosidic bindings between N-acetylglucosamine and asparagine.

Functional Aspects

Little is known about the physiological role of Kt-PG. In the second part of life it increases in quantity, in step with collagen and chondroitin-6-sulfate. Patients with macular corneal dystrophy are not able to form any mature Kt-PG (*Hascall* et al. 1980).

Structural Glycoproteins

Collagen

Synthesis, molecular and supramolecular structure

With the exception of the blood cells, all cell types, at least up to a certain level of development, seem to be capable of collagen synthesis (*Hay* overview, 1980).

It is difficult to ignore the genetic control of collagen synthesis; apart from the genes, that determine the primary structure simultaneously genes have to code for enzymes with functions that include controlling the correct length of the triple-helical molecule, its glycosylation, cross-meshing and polymerization in the cell, as well as the extracellular egestion of the procollagen molecule (tropocollagen). GAGs and PGs are determinants for extracellular maturation to collagen fibrils (Fig. 6).

Intracellular biosynthesis of collagen includes the following steps: the amino acid sequence of the three individual α-chains (primary structure) of the triple helical molecule in the various collagen-producing cells is determined by the formation of corresponding messenger-RNA at the responsible DNA sections of certain chromosomes (human chromsomes 7 and 17 for type 1 procollagen of the cornea and the human skin; overview in *Hay* 1980). (400,000 basic pairs of DNA are determined for the pro-α_2 gene; it contains about 60 exons [coded regions], that are interrupted by introns [non-coded sequences]). Corresponding to the DNA message, procollagen molecules are assembled from pro-α-chains at the ribosomes of the endoplasmic reticulum under temporary addition of transfer-RNA molecules (each of which brings the appropriate amino acid). It appears that "signal peptides" at the end of the procollagen molecules make penetration of the ribosomes into the tube system of the endoplasmic reticulum ("pre-collagen") possible. They are removed as they cross the membrane. The helix formation of the α-chains follows up to the Golgi apparatus, the terminal and packing station of the endoplasmic reticulum, i.e. the bringing together of 3 α-chains to the triple helix (tertiary structure; Fig. 6). The 3 α-chains are wound around one another and form a super-helix, apart from the non-helical COOH and NH_2 ends.

Hydrogen-bridge bindings inside and between the individual α-chains are involved in the development of the secondary and tertiary structures. Glycine has a special role in the formation and stabilisation of this binding. It forms the third amino acid along each α-polypeptide chain. Hydroxylysine has a special influence on the stability of the triple helix formation, replacing approximately every hundredth proline as enzymatic hydroxylated proline (*Hay* 1980). It is important that proline and lysine are only one third hydroxylated as they are built-in to the α-chain, or one sixth through an enzyme system (co-factors are present: oxygen, ascorbic acid, α-ketoglutarate and iron (Fe^{2+} ions). At the same time, some of the hydroxyl groups of the hydroxylysine are attached to galactosyl-glucose or galactose groups. Collagen is thus a glycoprotein, and functionally it is a structural glycoprotein. The large amounts of the amino acids, glycine (23–29%), proline (15–16%) and hydroxyproline (11–14%) stand out. Glycine and the amino acids repeating themselves at every third site are important for regular helical folding (abot 333 glycine remnants per chain).

The α-chains thus consist of a sequence of amino acid triplets of the Gly-X-Y type. Either X or Y can be an amino acid. The commonest (in about 100 triplets on an α-chain) are, however, X-proline and Y-hydroxyproline (Hay 1980). Out of 1.000 amino acid remnants, 81 are charged positively and 82 negatively, i.e. collagen is almost electrically neutral (for piezoelectricity, see below and the contribution by *Bergsmann*).

The formation of an α-chain lasts about 10 minutes. The total synthesis of a molecule, including egestion, lasts 35 to 40 minutes (*Olsen* 1983). Extracellularly, the triple-helical collagen molecule is about 280 nm long, with a diamter of 1,5 nm. The triple helix structure is stabel at 37°C, but above 40°C it begins to unfold (*Harkness* 1970). During egestion into the extracellular space, the non-helical telopeptides at the COOH and NH_2 ends are partly split off by a procollagen protease. The telopeptides are bound together by disulfide bridges and intermeshed through glycolized hydroxylysine. The telopeptides thus contribute to the intracellular stability of the procollagen molecules and prevent premature fibril formation. The telopeptides parts split off during egestion act as negative feedback inhibitors of collagen synthesis. Since the terminal intermeshings appear outside the triple helix configuration, they are much more accesible to proteolysis than before. Finally, only collagenases from macrophages and neutrophilic granulocytes can attack the extremely stable collagen molecule (*Hay* 1980).

The linearly-arranged molecules overlap one another at the ends by about 27 nm, i.e. a quarter of the length of the molecule (Fig. 6). There is a cavity region about 40 nm in diameter between the staggered collagen molecules, between the COOH head and the NH_2 end. The glycosyl derivates of the cavity region are not only participants in the intermeshing of the collagen molecules, they have, among other functions, that of binding water and exchanging cations, so that the "start region" in ossification processes lays in the cavity sections, through addition and storage of hydroxylapatite crystals (overview in *Hay, Linsenmayer 1983).*

Collagen Modification

Since hydroxylysine and hydroxyproline are present in the collagen molecule in varying amounts, and their glycolysis also varies, there are a great many modifications of the collagen molecule. Varying types of messenger RNA, as well as the disulfide groups of the telopeptides also

cause certain differences in molecular construction. At the moment, 5 biochemically and functionally different types of collagen molecule are differentiated (*Linsenmayer* 1983).
1. The collagen molecule with two α-1-chains and one α-2-chain has the widest distribution in connective tissue, including bone and dentin. It is termed Type I collagen and written with the formular [α1 (I)]-α2(I).
2. Type II collagen, mainly found in cartilage, consists of three identical α1-chains; correspondingly, the formula is: [α1(II)]3. Type I and Type II collagen can polymerize in the same fibrils, as was shown in the corneas of chickens.
3. Type III collagen is an important structural glycoprotein, which interlaces the extracellular matrix as a fine "reticular" network. It consists of 3α1-chains. Formula:[α1(III)3. Type III collagen contains a very large amount of 4-hydroxyproline and glycine, as well as 2 cystine remnants per α-chain.
4. Type IV collagen is a part of basement membranes. There are non-helical regions in the molecule (*Kefaldis*1978).
5. Type V collagen is also limited to the basement membranes, and is particularly easily attacked by collagenase from tumor cells.

Up to now, knowledge of these collagen types has made a significant contribution to the explanation of connective tissue diseases (e.g. Marfan syndrome, osteogenesis imperfecta, chondrodystrophy).

In side-to side polymerization of tropocollagen molecules to fibrils, typical striations with 12 bands appear in positive contrasting using phosphotungstic acid, from about 10 nm. These correspond to polar sections, and the interspaces to apolar regions in a microfibril. This arrangement is connected with the approximately $^1/_4$ displacement of the molecules in the primary fibrils. Up to repetition, the periodicity is about 67 nm (Fig. 6). The biological half-life varies between 1 and 630 days (*Olsen* 1983). The fibrils (diameter 10–25 nm) aggregate to fibers (diameter about 0.3 μm), and these to fiber bundles several millimeters thick (Fig. 6). Broken-down tropocollagen bundles are always found in the extracellular matrix, and these can contribute to growth in the thickness of the fiber bundles (Fig. 6). It can be precipitated by amino acids (e.g. valine from bacteria). Under pathological conditions, end-to-end and head-to-head bindings with periodicity of up to 280 nm (long-spacing collagen) can also appear (Fig. 6).

Functional Aspects

The thickness of the collagen fibrils is organ-specific and changes with age. Non-enzymatic glycosilation with a tendency to ion and lipoprotein binding plays a major role in the ageing process of collagen.

Tendons have collagen fibrils arranged in the longitudinal axis, and thus have, for example, only a tenth of the tensile strength of skin with its fiber bundles running in all directions. Here, quality plays a major role: tendons are made of Type I collagen; all types of collagen are found in skin. In addition, there is an initial arrangement of the fibers in the tension direction before the individual fibers are subjected to stress.

A two-phase system arises through the sugar binding on the tropocollagen molecule (mainly in the area of cavities, see above) and association of proteoglycans of the extracellular matrix on the surfaces of fibrils and fibers (*Henle's* sheath). Inter alia, this is mainly capable of water binding, which leads to stabilization and orientation of the fibers. Owing to low elasticity, relative tensile strength and a higly asymmetrical length-breadth relationship, collagen makes a significant contribution to the viscosity of the extracellular matrix, apart from GAGs and PGs. Globular molecules show this effect in dissimilarly small quantity. This is easy to recognize when a collagen solution which is still lying in natural asymmetry in the molecule is warmed above the denaturing temperatur of collagen (> 40°C). The viscosity of the solution then reduces rapidly, and only reappears when the temperature is lowered below this level.

The antigenicity of the collagen types is relatively low, and tyrosine may play a leading role (*Schmitt* et al. 1964, *Linsenmayer* 1983). Procollagen shows a higher antigenicity than tropocollagen (Overview in *Olsen* 1983). A highly significant property of collagen, that has been given little attention up to now, is its piezoelectrical property (*Athenstaedt* 1969; contribution by *Bergsmann*).

Under this one understands electrical charges appearing in deformation under mechanical demands (pressure, tension, torsion).

As *Athenstaedt* (1969) showed, piezoelectrical power already plays an important role at the stage of arrangement and polymerization to fibrils of the tropocollagen molecules egested from the fibroblasts. However, permanent electrical polarization does not only appear in the longitudinal axis of a collagen fiber, it also appears at right angles. The electrical polarization in the longitudinal axis is simple to explain: it concerns the fact that the tropocollagen molecule is morphologically asymmetrical. The polar and apolar amino acids are distributed asymmetrically along the axis of the molecule. Some carry an excess of positive charges, and others an excess of negative charges. The charge center does not coincide with the molecular axis; it is a certain distance away from there. As a result the tropocollagen molecule behaves like a dipole, with one direction in the molecular axis and the other at right angles to it. The single-axis optical double refraction of the collagen fibril corresponds to this. On the other hand, it is difficult to explain the permanent electrical polarization at right angles to the course of the fibril. According to *Athenstaedt* (1969), this is not coupled to the influence of adjacent tissue or to the direction of veering-out collagen fibrils. However, the hexagonal packing of collagen fibrils inside a fiber is too strong for a piezoelectric effect to result. It was also thought that the proteoglycans built into the fibrils could cause the effect. However, in bones dating from the ice age, it could be shown that the same piezoelectricity was present, although the protoglycans were long destroyed. The reason for the electrical polarization of collagen at right angles to the fiber axis therefore has to lie in the ultrastructure of the collagen molecule itself. Hexagonal packing of the tropocollagen molecule appears in the apolar region of a microfibril. In the polar regions, with the amino acids glutamine, asparagine, lysine and arginine, there is no hexagonal packing. Correspondingly, there is no marked electrical polarization at these sites. The intermeshing of tropocollagen molecules is, however, brought about to a significant extent by the chemically active side-chains of the polar amino acids. The electrical polarization at right angles to the longitudinal fiber axis could be bound to these side-chains, if one assumes – and there are findings available on this (radiological structural analysis, double refraction of swollen collagen fibers) – that they are arranged along the fibril axis in such a way that there is no rotation symmetry, and the positive charges are mainly on the one side, with an excess of negative charges mainly on the opposite side. At the same time, this means that the strength and quantity of the cross-networks on one side of the microfibril have to be greater than those on the other side (*Athenstaedt* 1969)! An important consequence of this is, for example, that in fracture healing, the cells of callus tissue and the adjacent bone are obviously able to "understand" this electrical potential pattern via their cell membranes, and regulate the reconstruction of the supporting structures accordingly.

Elastin

Synthesis, molecular and supramolecular structure

Synthesis follows the same principles as those described for collagen. Here too, fibroblasts and smooth muscle cells of the vascular wall are capable of elastin synthesis. A soluble proelastin (tropoelastin) is released into the extracellular space, and aggregates to insoluble elastin fibrils through cross-networks. These mature to branched fibers that only carry a sugar coating on their surfaces (*Heine* and *Schaeg* 1979, Fig. 1). Elastin does not contain any neutral sugars, hexosamine, cystine or tryptophan (*Franzblau* and *Faris* 1983).

Similar to the type Gly-X-Y amino acid triplets that repeat themselves in the collagen molecule, protoelastin contains the Gly-Val-Pro-Gly tetrapeptide. Alterations in the sequence lead to appropriate differences in the elastin molecule. However, the high glycine and hydroxyproline content could be an indication that elastin may be able to develop from collagen (*Heine* and *Schaeg*, 1979).

During the extracellular maturation process of tropoelastin, which, in contrast to collagen maturation, tends to be inhibited by ascorbic acid, there is development of desmosin and isodesmosin, the typical amino acids of elastin. They consist of lysine cross-networks. Initially, deamination of the lysine amino group through lysil oxidase leads to lysine aldehyde (allysine). (All agents that interfere with this step hinder the formation of the cross-network, e.g. D-penicillamin or the Lathryogen β-aminoproprionitril). With aldehyde remnants of the same or adjacent tropoelastin molecules, allysine can be accompanied by aldol condensation, and this leads to desmosin. Alternatively, non-oxidized lysine can form a *Schiff's* base with allysine via its amino group, leading to the formation of isodesmosin. Desmosin and isodesmosin form the sugar-free nuclei of elastic fibers. However, there are glycosylized microfibrils around the amorphous center (diameter about 8 nm). In contrast to amorphous elastin, these microfibrils have a high cystine content (70 to 80 cystine remnants per 1.000 amino acids). The numerous cystine-disulfide bridges that result are responsible for the relative insolubility of the microfibrils. According to *Scherr* et al., (1970), the amino acid sequence of the microfibrils has a remarkable agreement with the terminal NH_2 and COOH chains of the protocollagen molecules. The microfibrils have an influence on the orientation and form of the maturing fibers, and thus on the formation of the cross-networks. Hydroxyproline, hydroxylysine and lysine do not take part in the cross-networking process (*Franzblau* and *Faris* 1983).

Special, immature, very fine elastic fibrils (diameter about 8–10 nm) are termed oxytalan fibers; they support the anchoring of basement membranes in the extracellular matrix. With Type III collagen, oxytalan fibers form the optically visible part of the basement membrane. The mat-like weaving of Type III collagen and oxytalan fibers also covers the parenchymal cells as a fiber stocking, and thus retains them in "form" at the microscopic level.

Functional Aspects

Among other functions, elastic fibers are the basis of the flexibility and normal tone of the skin, lungs and blood vessels. Like collagen, elastin has its highest functional capacity, i.e. rubberlike flexibility, at 37°C. It was shown by experiment that elastin takes on a glass-like consistency at 20°C, and becomes brittle (review: *Franzblau* and *Faris* 1983). According to *Hoeve* (1977), lipid deposits in the vessel walls bring the "glass point" to the region of 37°C. Elastic fibers can be stretched up to 130% of their initial length, which is 20–30 times more than collagen. Elastic fibers form three-dimensional networks that are not affected by heat, acids or alkalis. With ageing, they diminish in number, particularly in the arterial walls in arteriosclerotic change.

Elastin is broken down more easily than collagen by trypsin and pepsin. Elastases were isolated from neutrophil granulocytes, macrophages, thrombocytes and pancreatic tissue (*Olsen* review 1983).

However, these enzymes are non-specific. While cellular elastase has a high proteolytic activity for leucylpeptide bindings, pancreatic elastase has high specificity for adenylpeptide bindings.

Excessive elastolytic activity appears, for example, in pulmonary emphysema, pancreatitis and arteriosclerosis (*Franzblau* and *Faris* 1983). The proteolytic enzymes bromealin, papain, ficin, pronase and nagase also attack elastic fibers (*Franzblau* 1971).

The relationships between elastin and collagen determine the mechanical capacity of connective tissue. The typical undulation of collagen fibers is attained through the irregular, spiral investment by elastic fiber networks. Tension-traction diagrams of normal elastic fibers show a point from which there is a sudden increase in the values for tensile power.

Morphologically, this can be understood as an arrangement of the elastic fiber networks along the collagen fibers, with their undulations acting as a reserve. The time-dependence of this process gives a standard for the viscoelasticity of the tissue. At the same time, this is a measurement of conformation changes in the macromolecules, with possibilities for intermolecular displacement (review: *Franzblau* and *Faris* 1983).

Irregular conformation changes are described for mucopolysaccaridoses: in Marfan's syndrome, for example, major differences from the normal tension-traction curve relationships appear in the aortic wall in the longitudinal and transverse directions (*Yamada* 1970).

Through this, pathological states such as aneurysms, dissecting aneurysm, dilatation of the aortic valves, and others, can appear. In principle, it is to be assumed that all pathological changes in the extracellular matrix are accompanied by changes in the conformation of its macromolecules.

From the energy point of view, a higher state of order means a reduction of entropy (random molecule distribution). Reduced order is thus accompanied by an increase in entropy, which means major construction and direction deformation possibilities for fibrillar molecules.

Gosline (1976) discussed whether energy could be stored through the interaction (Coulomb charges) of hydrophobic groups of elastic fibers with water molecules during stretching. It can be assumed that Coulomb charges play a significant role in the maintenance of the collagen – elastin – PG – GAG binding, and its viscoelastic behaviour, due to interactions with water molecules.

The elastic fibers differ qualitatively and quantitatively in the various tissues (*Olsen* review 1983): in cattle, the nuchal ligament is 80% elastin; the fibers are very thick (6.7 μm) and consist of short, rod-shaped fibers. In elastic arteries the elastin content is about 50%. In contrast, in skin, loose connective tissue and tendons, elastin makes up 5% to 2% of the dry weight. About 50 to 60 elastic membranes are arranged in concentric layers in the tunica media of the human aorta. They are 2.5 μm thick, and separated by 6–18 μm broad connective tissue spaces filled with extracellular matrix, which contains smooth muscle cells and frameworks of collagen and elastic fibers.

Network-forming Glykoproteins

Currently, we differentiate between fibronectin, laminin and chondronectin. The common factor between these high-molecular, sialinized glycoproteins is that they mediate between cell surfaces and the extracellular matrix due to their collagen binding capacity, and are exceptionally easy to split by proteolysis (review in *Yamada* 1983 and in *Haynes* 1983).

Fibronectin

The molecule was discovered on the cell surface (*Haynes* lit. 1983), then found as "tissue adhesive" in the extracellular matrix, and finaly recognized as an important constituent of blood plasma (300 μg/ml). It was also shown in the cerebrospinal fluid (3 μg/ml) and the amniotic fluid (60–80 μg/ml). Fibronectin appears to be formed by all cell types apart from erythrocytes and lymphocytes, particularly fibrocytes, macrophages, granulocytes and epithelial cells. It appears at a very early stage of embryonic development, and has been shown in mice in the morula stage (*Toole* 1983).

As a monomer molecule, tissue fibronectin has a molecular weight of 220.000–240.000 D, and a carbohydrate content of 5%. It appears as a monomeric, dimeric and polymeric molecule (Fig. 7). Fibronectin is found dissolved in plasma as a dimeric molecule. The fibronectin subunits are highly asymmetrical. No α-helical or β-folded bindings have been observed. The molecule is constructed from polypeptide domains, bound by folded-round polypeptide chains. They can stretch or shorten themselves, according to the ion relationships in their environment. Five sugars bound to asparagine appear at each monomer molecule (N-acetylglucosamine, mannose, galactose, fucose, sialinic acid). The oligosaccharide chains mark the collagen-binding and cell-binding part of the molecule. The half-life of fibronectin, like that of protein, is generally 30–36 hours. The fibronectin molecule has a variety of molecule-specific binding sites (Fig. 7): there is a collagen-binding part near the carboxyl end. The cell-surface-binding part lies between this and the amino (NH_2) end of the molecule. This includes binding sites for heparan sulfate, heparin-, hyaluronic acid- and proteoglycans. Between the heparin- (heparan sulfate) and collagen-binding part there is an actin-binding area. This has special significance since findings are available which show that fibronectin can appear transmembranously, connected to the actin of the microfilament bundles of the cytoskeleton. Cytochalasin A and B, which can destroy the microfilament system in cytoplasm, lead to a separation of the fibronectin bound to the cell surfaces (*Yamada* 1983).

Functional Aspects

Fibronectin is involved in all cellular growth, differentiation and movement processes. It also mediates cell adhesion to basement membranes, which leads to prevention of reciprocal cell migration (tumor cells do not have this contact inhibition). Fibronectin intermeshes the macromolecules of the extracellular matrix with one another and with the glycocalyx of cell surfaces. Through the enzyme transglutaminase (Blood coagulation factor XIII), fibronectin can be cross-meshed covalently intravasally and extravasally, which can also lead to the formation of complexes with collagen and fibrils (*Hay* overview 1980).

Since fibronectin can form a transmembranous binding to the cytoplasmic microfilament system (cytoskeleton) with its actin-binding

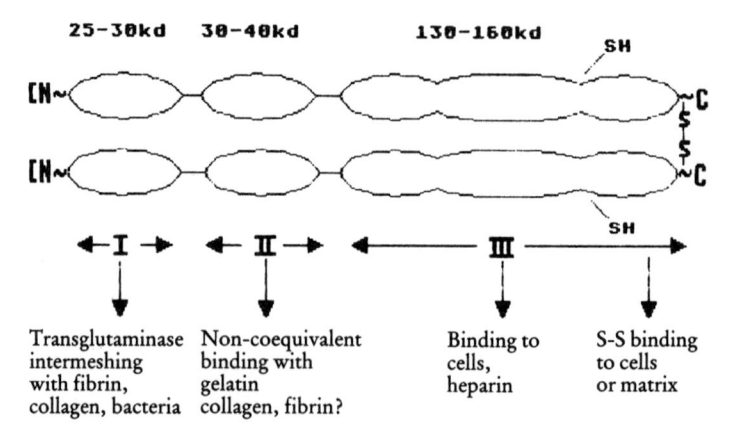

Fig. 7: Diagram of the structure of fibronectin. The dotted line regions can be split by pepsin. Each arm is about 2 nm in diameter, and contains larger globular parts at its end (about 5-7 nm) (from *Martin* and *Yamada* 1983).

area, this leads to numerous extra-intracellular (and vice versa) information pathways, which make rapid reactions by the cells and cell groups to changes in homeostasis possible. In contrast, tumor cells show an irregular cytoskeleton. Accordingly characteristic features appear in glycocalyx formation and fibronectin binding, which can make reciprocal recognition difficult for these cells, and leads to loss of contact inhibition. Due to the high proteolytic sensitivity of fibronectin, the informative coupling between the cells and the extracellular matrix can be severely disturbed through a non-physiological increase in proteases (e.g. all types of inflammation, shock, rheumatic disease). However, the sugar content of fibronectin prevents a too rapid proteolytic splitting and too rapid turnover of the polypeptide chains (*Yamada* 1983, *Heine* and *Domann* 1984).

It can be shown in animal experiments that there is intravascular and extravascular diminution of fibronectin by proteolysis within 10 minutes of a traumatic shock event, which leads to a general cellular alarm reaction (*Heine* and *Domann* 1984). On the other hand, it can be observed in embryonic myotubes that fibronectin is needed in the alteration of myotubes to striated muscle fibers. In further development, fleck-like fibronectin areas remain on the muscle fiber plasma membranes; they seem to be the start-point for the development of myoneural synapses (motor end-plates) (overview in *Sengbush* 1980). Among other points in favour of this is the fact that acetyl cholinesterase, which breaks down the neurotransmitter acetylcholine in the myoneural synapses, shows a collagen-related endpart. It could therefore be possible that the enzyme binds to the muscle fiber surfaces in the region of the postsynaptic membrane section via fibronectin, and becomes correspondingly effective in information transmission, or contributes to the development and renewal of this type of synapse. Since proteoglycans and fibronectin appear together in the extracellular matrix, and certain PGs are also direction determinants for the growth of nerve fibers, fibronectin seems to be involved in directional control and the growth of axons in the central nervous system as well as in the periphery (overview in *Sengbush* 1980, overview in *Toole* 1983).

In the plasma and extracellular matrix, fibronectin also has the function of an "opsonin" for antigens: i.e. after binding of fibronectin to the antigen surface, this is recognized as foreign by macrophages and neutrophilic granulocytes, and ingested and destroyed by phagocytosis. Since complement factor C1q has a collagen-related terminal part, it also becomes an opsonin after binding to fibronectin. It is significant that the actin-binding region of fibronectin can also bind DNA. If this is released from broken-down cells in large amounts (including tumors and shock), it can be opsonized through firbronectin, and rendered harmless (*Yamada* 1983). Fibronectin has special functions when there is destruction of vascular endothelium. First of all, thrombocytes cover the defect, and while doing so give off a series of substances that lead to the binding of further platelets. The coagulation cascade is stimulated, with local fibrin deposition, and an insoluble thrombus is formed under enzymatic net-formation through transglutaminase (from thrombocytes?) with fibrin. Here, the fibrin sources are by the plasma, the endothelial basement membrane and broken-down endothelial cells. Endothelial cells have little fibronectin on the side facing the lumen, but a great deal of heparin. Even against a gradient of 100:1, endothelial cells can pump heparin from the extracellular matrix at their surfaces (*Jacques* 1980). As a result, the endothelial side facing the lumen has a strong negative charge, and this raises its antithrombotic effect even more (*Heine* 1986). On the other hand, fibronectin can aggregrate heparin to fibrils, thus supporting thrombus formation (*Hynes* 1983).

Laminin

This glycoprotein is limited to the basement membranes. According to *Timpl* et al. (1978), laminin consists of two polypeptide chains, each with a molecular weight of 220,000 D. The two chains are bound to one another by disulfide bridges. The carbohydrate content is about 20%, and 4–6% of this is sialic acid. The macromolecule consists of one long and three short arms, with globular endings (Fig. 8). Laminin is not formed by fibrocytes.

The main sources are epithelia and striated muscle fibers. Functionally, laminin is mainly involved in the adhesion of epithelia to the collagen of the basement membrane (Type IV). It also binds to heparin and heparan sulfate, which are constituents of the basement membranes (overview in *Hynes* 1983).

Chondronectin

Hewitt et al. (1980) discovered this glycoprotein (molecular weight about 180,000 D) in cartilage and serum. In mesenchymal tissue in transition to cartilage formation, chondronectin is replaced by fibronectin.

Functionally, chondronectin is an adhesion factor for chondrocytes at cartilagineous collagen (Type II) (Overview in *Hynes* 1983).

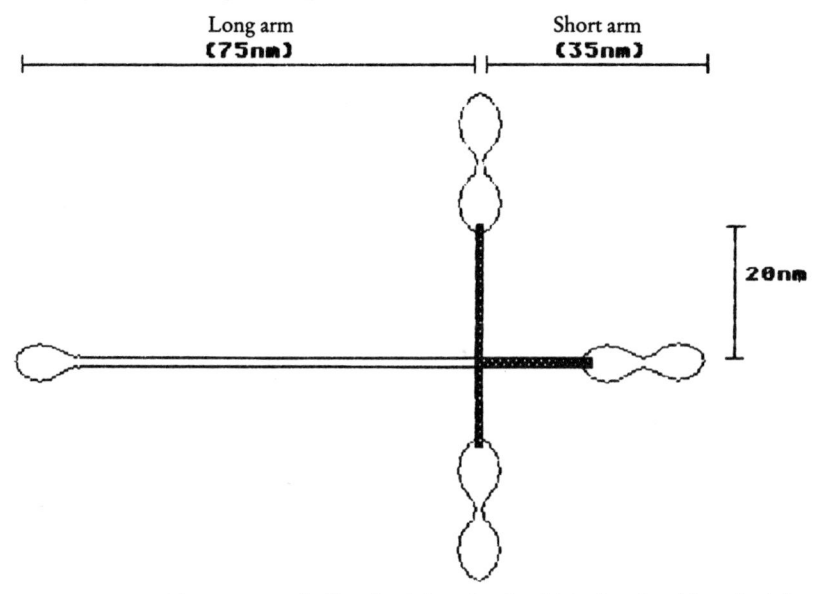

Fig. 8: Diagram of the structure of a dimer laminin molecule with its functional domains (after *Hynes* 1983)

Energy flow in the Extracellular Matrix

Demonstration of the functional morphology of the extracellular matrix can emphasize certain, logically-based forms of life, but without making the prime mover any clearer. The common denominator of all biological reactivity lies in its energy flow. The material basics of biological energy are the various sugar biopolymers, water, the substances dissolved in it, and their proportions in the structure. Biological energy is quantitatively and qualitatively tangible as biodynamics (quality transformation between energy and mass). A very clear example of this is the interaction between water and the extracellular matrix; the energy flow between the molecular swarms of liquid-crystaline water and the sugar molecules determine the degree of organization and thus the structural proportions in the extracellular matrix.

Since all vital functions are mediated by the extracellular matrix, it may not have a higher energy consumption than superior specialized systems such as cells and cell groups. Since the extracellular matrix is a dissipative system, whose states of organization are not stable, oscillating far from thermodynamic stability, spontanous reactions in the extracellular matrix are, with the production of new patterns and arrangements that spread themselves by autocatalysis, the expression of life-retaining ground interactions and quality transformations between energy and mass. The processes appear spontaneoulsy when the free energy of the products is lower than that of the reactants.

The free energy exchange of a system (G) shows the sum of all kinetic and potential energy factors (this is termed enthalpy H). The temperature-dependent alterations (T) of the random distribution of the participating molecules (so-called entropy (S). The result is the following formula:

$$\Delta G = \Delta H - T\Delta S \qquad (1)$$

The kinetic energy that appears is primary translational (E_t) and rotational (E_r). Translation energy corresponds to the collision between the macromolecules, which can be made visible as *Brownian* movement. For two macromolecules to be able to react with one another they have to assume a specific conformation status through rotational energy.

With the correct relationship to each other molecules can enter into two forms of binding, without reduction of their potential energy: a) covalent bindings; they reduce the potential energy by about 100 Kcal/mol, and b) secondary bindings (*v.d. Waalsian* charges) with a reduction of only about 5 Kcal/mol. Secondary bindings have greater significance in the extracellular matrix. They include: a) dispersive bindings. They appear with the attraction of two non-polar atoms. The reduction of potential energy is 0.05 to 0.2 Kcal/mol. Hydrophobic bindings also belong here (*Coulombian* charges); these are brought about by water, as very weak dispersive bindings. The information from *Gosline* (1976) can be used as an example, namely that it appears that elastic energy can be stored during stretching of the fibers due to interaction of the hydrophobic groups of the elastic fibers with water molecules, and can be given off as the fibers return to their original state; b) electrostatic bindings. They can attract and repel, and thus reduce or increase the potential energy. Hydrogen bridges that mediate between two atoms are of major significance as electrostatic bindings for the energy system in the extracellular matrix.

Potential energy is thus either covalently (P_c) electrostatically (P_E) or dispersively (P_D) effectice in the extracellular matrix, although the kinetic energy appears primarily translationally (E_t) and rotationally (E_r). The sum of the energy factors in the extracellular matrix (enthalpy) is thus summarized as follows:

$$H = P_C + P_E + P_D + E_t + E_r \tag{2}$$

$$\Delta H = \Delta G + T \Delta S \tag{3}$$

$$\Delta S = k \ln(N)$$
$$k = Boltzmann \text{ constant} \tag{4}$$

According to (1) and (3), the enthalpy (ΔH) of the extracellular matrix corresponds to the energy exchange of the system (ΔG) and its proportion of entropy (ΔS). Entropy is proportional to the conformation status of macromolecules and the number of spatial positions (N) that can be taken-in by a small molecule like water. Entropy is thus accompanied by structural breakdown and enthalpy by structural formation.

If the conformtion possibilities of molecules increase, or the volume occupied by a molecule grows (e.g. due to heating), then, in accordance with (3) this corresponds to an increase in entropy, through which the net quantity of free energy decreases, in accordance with (1). Interactions in the extracellular matrix can thus be predominantly entropy-reducing or predominantly enthalpy-reducing. As the molecular sieve between capillaries and cells, both systems must be nearly in balance in the organization of the extracellular matrix. If the enthalpy share is too great, the result is an excessive increase in entropy, and the result is that the macromolecular system of order is lost (acute diseases, inflammation, allergies, rheumatic diseases, neoplasms). If there is too little free exchange of energy, entropy is destroyed, and the result is the development of super-molecular states of order that are also not compatible with normal function of the extracellular matrix (scleroses, nodules, sarcoma).

The balance between enthalpy and entropy is extremely labile and is thus easily influenced by energy. It is, however, the precondition for the retention of all molecular order in a biological flow balance. In contrast to closed-energy systems (*Newtonian* systems), the labile balance of molecular interactions in an open-energy system does not lead to random molecular collision, but to spontaneous, always new, interdependent states of order with self-catalytic capacities. Spontaneity should therefore not be confused with chance. Spontaneity is always only possible in states of order that are labile. The random molecular collisions in closed systems finally lead to thermodynamic balance (e.g. the temperature adjustment in a piece of red-hot iron placed in a bucket of cold water). For open-energy systems this stable balance would be the same as their destruction; i.e. there is no "chance" in living systems. The preconditions and retention of all life is bound to the spontaneity of molecular interactions in an open-energy system. This is also the basis of all biorhythms. A "fatal" thermodynamic balance can only be prevented in this way.

Basically, all culture is concerned with influencing the spontaneity of biomolecular interactions in the extracellular matrix through life-style. From the molecular point of view, the task of medicine is thus the maintenance of the individual spontaneity of molecular interactions within the framework of homeostasis.

The extremely low energy charges that suffice to initiate spontaneous reactions in biological systems reflect an experience principle that has its roots in the medicine of ancient times, namely that a highly diluted poison can be a healing substance. That is, that a substance that destroys the spontaneity of molecular biological reactions can support these reactions if its reaction capacity is reduced to the level of the reaction between water and sugar biopolymers.

This principle was revived by *Paracelsus* for academic medicine, and finally taken into the science of homeopathy in the 19th century through *Hahnemann* with the motto "similia similibus currentur". The "simile" principle, according to which similar can be healed by similar, is a treatment indication for the molecular biology principle of spontaneous reactions in the open-energy system extracellular matrix. Naturally, cells are also an open-energy system, but their switching-on always follows that of the extracellular matrix.

Homeopathy is thus, unlike any other experience-medicine discipline, directed towards the molecular interactions and transformations between sugar biopolymers and liquid-crystalline water. Since the spontaneity of these interactions is already the expression of individuality, it can be understood that a precise case history, including the biographic and social history, is extremely important for the physician using homeopathic methods. Only then can the "simile" principle be effective. The drugs diluted according to this principle are suitable for stimulating the spontaneous autocatalytic reactivity of ground regulation, and, when used correctly, for restoring it to its individual proportions. Here, it can be particularly important that the greatest dilutions, that do not contain any molecules of the initial substance in the solvent (alcohol, water), have a structurally-caused energy content due to the dilution process, which, as experience shows, can suffice for allaying complaints, and can also bring healing. Here, from the molecular biology point of view, the spontaneity of extracellular matrix reactivity can be stimulated in an appropriate way. Homeopathy is thus a medical discipline that is directed towards stimulation and restoration of the individual biodynamics and bioenergy of ground regulation according to the "simile" principle.

Sugars – Witnesses of Precellular Evolution?

In the sugar biopolymers the significant elements seem to reflect precellular evolution: starting from carbohydrates, aldehydes and carbonic acid can be formed through simple oxidative steps. The latter can be altered to polysaccharides, proteins and fats through simple chemical reactions. According to the quantum chemistry investigations by *Goldanski* (1986), *Hoyle* and *Wickramasinghe* (1984), the development of polysaccharides is possible under the extreme conditions of interstellar (cosmic) space. The energy level needed for these types of reactions at normal temperatures does not need to be reached; it can be circumvented by quantum chemistry, i.e. the necessary energy requirement is under-tunneled (Fig. 9).

Tunnel processes permit chemical reactions at extremely low temperatures (*Goldanksi* 1986). As the researchers named showed, the interstellar formaldehyde demonstrable in this way has special significance, as was shown experimantally, it can close into chains of formaldehyde-polymers under these extreme conditions. Currently, the discussion is "whether interstellar formaldehyde molecules are really able to change themselves to stable polysaccharides like cellulose and starch" (*Goldanski* 1986). There is already evidence that quantum chemistry tunnel effects can also appear in

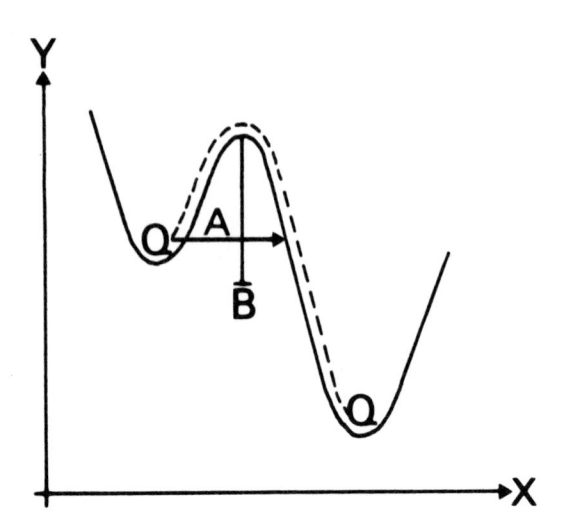

Fig. 9: Quantum chemistry tunnel processes between potential depressions (Q) permit chemical reactions that could not otherwise occur. Potential energy Y; reaction coordinate, spacing of atoms in molecule X. The interrupted line shows the normal activation barrier which needs activation energy (B) to be overcome. This barrier can be tunneled (A) with exceptionally low temperatures (from *Goldanski* 1986).

biopolymers at physiological temperatures (*Goldanski* 1986). It is strange that with this the natural philosophy ideas of *Giordano Bruno, Schelling* and *Goethe* on the cosmic ubiquity of the life principle receives support from the natural sciences, (in discussions with leading anthroposophic physicians, a consensus was reached that the ground regulation system is the morphological expression of the etheric body).

Literature

Abe, K., Sasaki, H., Takebayashi, K., Fukui, K., Nambu, H.: J. interdiscpl. Cycle Res. **9** (1978) 211 (zit. n. *Lemmer* 1983).

Ader, R.: Psychoimmuniology. Academie Press, New York, London 1981.

Athenstaedt, H.: Pyroelectric and piezoelectric properties of vertebrates. Ann. New York Acad. Sci. **238** (1974) 68–110.

Baker, J. H. and *Caterson, B.:* The isolation and characterization of the link proteins from proteoglycan aggregates of bovine nasal cartilage. J. Biol. Chem. **254** (1979) 2387–2393.

Balasz, E. A. and *Gibbs, P. A.:* The rheological properties and biological function of hyaluronic acid. In: *Balasz, E. A.* (Ed.): Chemistry and Molecular Biology of the Intercellular Matrix, Vol. 3. Academic Press, New York, London 1970, pp. 1241–1254.

Bergsmann, O. und *Bergsmann, R.:* Projektionssymptome. Reflektorische Krankheitszeichen als Grundlage für holistische Diagnose und Therapie. Facultas Universitätsverlag, Wien 1988.

Bertalanffy, L. V.: Perspectives of General System Theory. Braziller, New York 1975.

Bordeu, L.: Recherches sur le tissu muqueux ou l'organ cellulaire. Paris 1767.

Buddecke, E.: Grundriß der Biochemie. 2. Aufl. W. de Gruyter, Berlin 1971.

Buttersack, R.: Latente Erkrankungen des Grundgewebes, insbesondere der serösen Häute. Stuttgart 1912.

Cerami, A., Vlassara, H., Brownlee, M.: Glucose und Altern. Spektrum d. Wissenschaft 7 (1987) 44–51.

Chiarugi, V. P., Vanucchi, S., Cella, C., Fibbi, G., Delrosso, M., Capelletti, R.: Intercellular glycosaminoglycans in normal and neoplastic tissues. Cancer Res. **38** (1978) 4717–4725.

Christner, J. E., Brown, M. L., Dziewiatkowski, D. D.: Interactions of cartilage proteoglycans with hyaluronate. J. Biol. Chem. **254** (1979) 4624–4630.

Dorfman, A.: Proteoglycan Biosynthesis. In: *Hey, E.* (Ed.): Cell Biology of Extracellular Matrix. 2nd ed. Plenum Press, New York London 1983, pp. 115–138.

Dosch, J. P.: Lehrbuch der Neuraltherapie nach Huneke (Procain-Therapie). 5. Aufl. Karl F. Haug Verlag, Heidelberg 1975.

Engelberg, H.: Probable physiologic functions of heparin. Fed. Proc. **1** (1977), 36.

Eppinger, H.: Die Permeabilitätspathologie als die Lehre vom Krankheitsbeginn. Springer Verlag, Wien 1949.

Fintelmann, V.: Intuitive Medizin. Einführung in eine anthroposophisch ergänzte Medizin. 2. Aufl. Hippokrates Verlag, Stuttgart 1988.

Fischer, G.: Waschstumsdynamik und Bioenergetik. Messen, Steuern, Regeln (Berlin) **29** (1986) 98–100.

Franzblau, C. and *Raris, B.:* Elastin. In: *Hey, E. D.* (Ed.): Cell Biology of Extracellular Matrix. 2nd Ed. Plenum Press, New York, London 1983, pp. 65–94.

Fülgraff, G.: Der kontrollierte klinische Versuch – Eine kritische Würdigung. Pharmazeut. Ztg. **130** (1985) 3309–3313.

Goldanski, W. I.: Quantenchemische Reaktionen bei sehr tiefen Temperaturen. Spektrum d. Wissenschaft **4** (1986) 62–71.

Gosline, J. M.: The physical properties of elastic tissue. Int. Rev. Connect. Tissue Res. **7** (1976) 211–249.

Gutmann, V. und *Resch, G.:* Hochpotenz und Molekularkonzept. therapeutikon **4** (1988) 245–252.

Hascall, V.C. and *Hascall, G.K.:* Proteoglycans. In: *Hey, E.D.* (Ed.): Cell Biology of the Extracellular Matrix. 2nd Ed. Plenum Press, New York, London 1983, pp. 39–64.

Harkness, R.D.: Functional aspects of the connective tissue of skin. In: *Balasz, E.A.:* (Ed.): Chemistry and Molecular Biology of the Extracellular Matrix, Vol. 3. Academic Press, New York, London 1970.

Hauss, W.H., Junge-Hülsing, G., Gerlach, G.: Die unspezifische Mesenchymreaktion. Thieme, Stuttgart 1968.

Hay, E.D.: Extracellular Matrix. J. Cell Biol. **91** (1980) 205 s–223 s.

–, –: Collagen and Embryonic Development. In: *Hay, E.D.* (Ed.): Cell Biology of Extracellular Matrix. 2nd ed. Plenum Press, New York, London 1983, pp. 379–410.

Heine, H.: Vakuumprobleme bei histologischer Gefriertrocknung. G-I-T Fachz. f.d. Lab. Sonderheft Mai 1974, 531–532.

–, –: Basalmembranen als Regulationssystem zwischen epithelialen Zellverbänden. Gegenbaurs morph. Jahrb. **132** (1986) 325–331.

–, –: Die Grundregulation aus neuer Sicht. Ärztezeitschr. f. Naturheilverf. **28** (1987a) 909–914.

–, –: Regulationsphänomene der Tumorgrundsubstanz. Dtsch. Zschr. Onkol. **19** (1987b) 67–72.

–, –: Anatomische Struktur der Akupunkturpunkte. Dtsch. Zschr. Akup. **31** (1988a) 26–30.

–, –: Akupunkturtherapie – Perforationen der oberflächlichen Körperfaszie durch kutane Gefäß-Nervenbündel. therapeutikon **4** (1988b) 238–244.

–, –: Markierung von Blutzellen mit einem Lektin-Karbohydrat-Komplex. Erweiterte Funktionsdiagnostik an Blutausstrichen. Z. Mikrosk.-anat. Forsch. **102** (1988c) 54–62.

–, –: Grundregulation und Ganzheitsmedizin. Natur- und Ganzheitsmed. **3**, 1990 (a) 68–72.

–, –: Lehrbuch der biologischen Medizin. Hippokrates Verlag, Stuttgart 1990 (b)

–, – und *Henrich, H.:* Reactive behaviour of myocytes during long-term sympathetic stimulation as compared to spontaneous hypertension. Fol. Angiol. **28** (1980) 22–27.

–, – und *Schaeg, G.:* Informationssteuerung in der vegetativen Peripherie. Zschr. Hautkr. **54** (1979) 590–597.

–, – und *Domann, M.:* Fibronectin – plasmin-sensitive glycoprotein of the transit zone. Protetion by aprotinin. Arzneim.-Forsch./Drug Res. **34** (1984) 696–698.

Hewitt, A.T., Kleinmann, H.K., Pennpacker, J.P., Martin, G.R.: Identification of an adhesive factor for chondrocytes. Proc. Natl. Acad. Sci. USA **77** (1980) 385–388.

Hildebrandt, G.: Chronobiologische Untersuchungen autonomer Regulationen. Die Zeitstruktur hygiogenetischer Reaktionen. therapeutikon **1** (1987) 70–81.

Hobbs, H.: New Engl. J. Med **317** (1987) 734–737.

Hoeve, C.A.J. and *Flory, P.J.:* The elastic properties of elastin. Biopolymers **13** (1980) 677–686.

Hollemann, A.F. und *Richter, F.:* Lehrbuch der organischen Chemie, W. de Gruyter, Berlin 1964, S. 37–41.

Hoyle, F. and *Wickramasinghe, E.:* From Grains to Bacteria. University College Cardiff Press 1984.

Huneke, F.: Das Sekundenphänomen. 4. Aufl. Karl F. Haug Verlag, Heidelberg 1975.

Hynes, R.O.: Fibronectin and its relation to cellular structur and behavior. In: *Hay, E.D.* (Ed.): Cell Biology of Extracellular Matrix, 2nd ed. Plenum Press, New York, London 1983, pp. 295–334.

Iozzo, R.V.: Biology of Disease. Proteoglycans: Structure, Function, and Rol in Neoplasia. Lab. Invest. **53** (1985) 337–396.

Jaques, L.B.: Heparin: an old drug with a new paradigm. Science **206** (1979) 528–533.

Kefalides, N. A., Alper, R., Clark, C. C.: Biochemistry and metabolism of basement membranes. Int. Rev. Cytol. **61** (1979) 167–213.
Kellner, G. und *Kleine, G.:* Richtlinien zur Synovialzytologie. Z. f. Rheumatologie **35** (1976) 141–153.
König, W., Bohn, A., Theobald, K., Brehm, K. D., Knöller, J. J.: Die Mastzelle – zentraler Effektor bei allergischen Reaktionen. Klinikarzt **12** (1983) 753–776.
Lemmer, B.: Chronopharmakologie. Tagesrhythmen und Arzneimittelwirkung. Wissenschaftliche Verlagsgesellschaft, Stuttgart 1983.
Lenz, W.: Medizinische Genetik. 6. Aufl. Thieme Verlag, Stuttgart 1983.
Leupold, E.: Der Zell- und Gewebsstoffwechsel als innere Krankheitsbedingung. G. Thieme Verlag, Leipzig 1945.
–, –: Die Bedeutung des Blutchemismus besonders in Beziehung zu Tumorbildung und Tumorabbau. II. Teil. G. Thieme Verlag, Stuttgart 1954.
Levine, St. A. and *Kidd, M. P.:* Antioxidant Adaption. Its Role in Free Radical Pathology. Biocurrent Division, San Leandro, California 1985.
Linsenmeyer, T. F.: Collagen. In: *Hey, E. D.* (Ed.): Cell Biology of Extracellular Matrix. 2nd ed. Plenum Press, New York, London 1983, pp. 5–38.
Matthews, M. B.: Connective tissue. Macromolecular structure and evolution. Mol. Biol. Biochem. Biophys. **19** (1975) 1–318.
McBride, W. H. and *Bard, J. B.:* Hyaluronidase-sensitive halos around adherent cells. Their role in blocking lymphocyte-mediated phagocytosis. J. Exp. Med. **149**, 507–515.
Mohr, H.: Das Elementare in den Wissenschaften – Möglichkeiten und Grenzen des Reduktionismus. Vortrag zur Jahresversammlung „Das Elementare – Bestand und Wandel" der Deutschen Akademie der Naturforscher Leopoldina, Halle, 11. bis 14. 4. 1987. Nova Acta Leopold., NF (in Vorbereitung) zit. n. *Peil, J.:* Komplementarität von Kausalität und Finalität in der Biologie – ein rezensorischer Bericht über 2 Vorträge zur Jahresversammlung 1987 der Leopoldina. Gegenbaurs Morph. Jahrb. **134** (1988) 105–113.
Öbrink, B.: A study of the interactions between monomeric tropocollagen and glycosaminoglycans. Eur. J. Biochem. **33** (1973) 387–395.
Olsen, B. R.: Collagen Biosynthesis. In: *Hey, E. D.* (Ed.): Cell Biology of Extracellular Matrix. 2nd ed. Plenum Press, New York, London 1983, pp. 139–178.
Perger, F.: Die Vor- und Nachbehandlung von Herdsanierungen. natura-med. **1/2** (1987) 13–20 (1987) 68–75.
Pischinger, A.: Das Schicksal der Leukozyten. Z. mikr.-anat. Forsch. **63** (1957) 627–629.
–, –: Das System der Grundregulation. Grundlagen für eine ganzheitsbiologische Theorie der Medizin. 4. Aufl. Karl F. Haug Verlag, Heidelberg 1983.
Popp, F. A.: Neue Horizonte in der Medizin. Karl F. Haug Verlag, Heidelberg 1983.
Priebe, L.: Rhythmus des Lebendigen. Thermodynamik irreversibler Prozesse – dissipative Strukturen und Lebensvorgänge. Umschau **81** (1981) 43–48.
Psuya, P., Drouet, L., Zawilska, K.: Binding of heparin to human endothelial cell monolayer and extracellular matrix in culture. Thromb. Res. **47** (1987) 469–478.
Quincke, H.: Arch. exp. Path. Pharmak. **31** (1893) 211 (zit. n. *Lemmer* 1983).
Rapoport, S. M.: Medizinische Biochemie. 5. Aufl. VEB Volk und Gesundheit, Berlin 1969.
Ricker, G.: Pathologie als Naturwissenschaft. Springer Verlag, Berlin 1925.
Rindfleisch, E. v.: Elemente der Pathologie. Thieme Verlag, Leipzig 1869.
Rokitansky, C. v.: Handbuch der pathologischen Anatomie. Maudrich, Wien 1846.

Schmitt, F. O., Gross, J., Highberger, J. H.: Tropocollagen and the properties of fibrous collagen. Exp. Cell Res. Suppl. 3 (1955) 326–334.
Sengbusch, P. v.: Molekular- und Zellbiologie. Springer Verlag, Berlin, Heidelberg, New York 1979.
Sherr, C. J., Taubmann, M. B., Goldberg, B.: Isolation of a disulfide-stabilized, three-chain polypeptide fragment unique to the precursor of human collagen. J. Biol. Chem. **248** (1973) 7033–7038.
Stux, G.: Grundlagen der Akupunktur. 2. Aufl. Springer Verlag, Berlin, Heidelberg, New York 1988.

Takatsuki, A. and *Tamura, G.:* Effect of tunicamycin on synthesis of macromolecules in cultures of chick embryo fibroblasts infected with Newcastle disease virus. J. Antibiot. **24** (1977) 785–794.
Thomas, F.: Die Anwendung einfacher Prinzipien der Regelung komplexer Systeme auf die Humanmedizin. DEVLR-Mitt. 84–13, Braunschweig 1986.
Timpl, R., Martin, G. R., Bruckner, P., Wick, G., Wiedemann, H.: Nature of the collagenous protein in a tumor basement membrane. Eur. J. Biochem. **84** (1978) 43–52.
Toole, B. P.: Glycosaminoglycans in Morphogenesis. In: *Hey, E. D.* (Ed.): Cell Biology of Extracellular Matrix. 2nd ed. Plenum Press, New York, London 1983, pp. 259–294.
Trincher, K.: Die Gesetze der biologischen Thermodynamik. Urban u. Schwarzenberg Wien, München, Baltimore 1981.

Uhlenbruck, G., Beuth, H. J., Oette, K., Schotten, T., Ko, H. L., Roszkow, K., Roskowski, W., Lütticken, R., Pulverer, G.: Kektine und die Organotropie der Metastasierung. Dtsch. med. Wschr. 111 (1986) 991–995.

Wendt, L.: Die Eiweißspeicher-Krankheiten. Proteothesaurismosen. Karl F. Haug Verlag, Heidelberg 1984.
Wendt, L. und *Warning, H.:* Verschlackungs-Syndrome. Hufeland J. 2 (1986) 27–39.
Wiener, N.: Kybernetik – Regelung und Nachrichtenübermittlung im Lebewesen und in der Maschine, Econ-Verlag, Düsseldorf 1963.

Yamada, K. M.: Fibronectin and Other Structural Proteins. In: *Hey, E. D.* (Ed.): Cell Biology of Extracellular Matrix. 2nd ed. Plenum Press, New York, London 1983, pp. 95–114.

(Prof. Dr. rer. nat. med. habil. Hartmut Heine, Anatomisches Institut der Universität Witten/Herdecke, Dortmunder Landstr. 30, D-5804 Herdecke)

Part Two

The Ground System, Regulation and Regulatory Disturbances in Rehabilitation Practice

While the clinical picture of acute diseases is marked by massive pathomorphological changes and/or dangerous symptoms, these – apart from malignant processes and genetic defects – are both missing in patients with chronic diseases and illnesses. Here, dysfunctions and disturbances of health are in the foreground, whose cause is not immediately apparent. Mainly, the usual processes that provide a clinical picture, and the biochemical parameters are only found sparingly, or there is no reference point for possible therapy. The almost compulsory result is typical, false medical treatment; the diffuse, unclear condition is placed in the nearest clinical syndrome, and treated accordingly. *A chronic illness is changed into acute disease.*

The results of this mistake in thinking are known; and can be seen at any time in departments for the chronically ill or rehabilitation centers: in their usual doses, the drugs of acute medicine produce further regulation stress, and basically cannot combat the illness. This is even more true for operations (which are often not indicated). On the other hand, the additional iatrogenic regulatory stress from drugs leads to perpetuation and worsening of the illness.

However, there is no question of doubting the possibilities and the service provided by clinical medicine in acute, dangerous diseases and the field of emergency medicine. It should, however, be emphasized once again that the diagnostic and therapeutic methods of clinical medicine only have limited justification in chronic diseases, and then mainly in acute exacerbations.

The aim of diagnosis and therapy in chronic diseases have to be orientated to biocybernetic aspects and facts, also when regulation and/or dysregulation should be considered and treated with the usual clinical methods.

Physiological Regulatory Requirements

Before considering the problem of chronicity, it seems necessary to give a brief description of the facts of biocybernetics.

The organism – A Network System

The human organism, like every living organism, is an intermeshed, self-regulating system, and can thus, like other network systems, only be described through information flow, and not by mass or energy flow. Such self-regulatory systems are also, in principle, capable of oscillation.

It really does not need to be mentioned that the human system has to be regarded as a subsystem in relationship to the environment and the cosmos, and that it is constructed from further subsystems.

The Regulatory Cycle

The regulatory cycle is the smallest cybernetic unit. Here, it is only intended to serve as a basic description of the regulatory mechanisms, since it is not possible to observe the function of a single regulatory cycle in clinical medicine. But subsystems and systems that certainly can be observed react according to the same principles. It is also necessary to realize that the cyclic construction is not essential; the important point is the *cyclic function*. The task of this structure is to maintain *homeostasis*, and to correct deviations due to disturbances, with the minimal loss of energy. The latter also corresponds to the optimal coverage of requirements with the minimal loss of energy, namely a *principle of economy*.

The Functional Elements of the Regulatory Cycle are:

1. The *sensor*, with whose assistance the actual state in the measuring pathway is established, and transformed into signals that are transmitted to the regulator.

2. In the regulator the current state is compared with a a *guiding dimension,* mainly of external origin, and deviations between the *nominal value* and actual value are changed to signals, which are transmitted as *adjustment* values to the
3. *Adjustment arm.* The action of the adjustment arm now corrects the substrate measured by the sensor until the actuel value and nominal values agree.

It should be mentioned that there are sensors with various functions, such as differential, integral, etc.

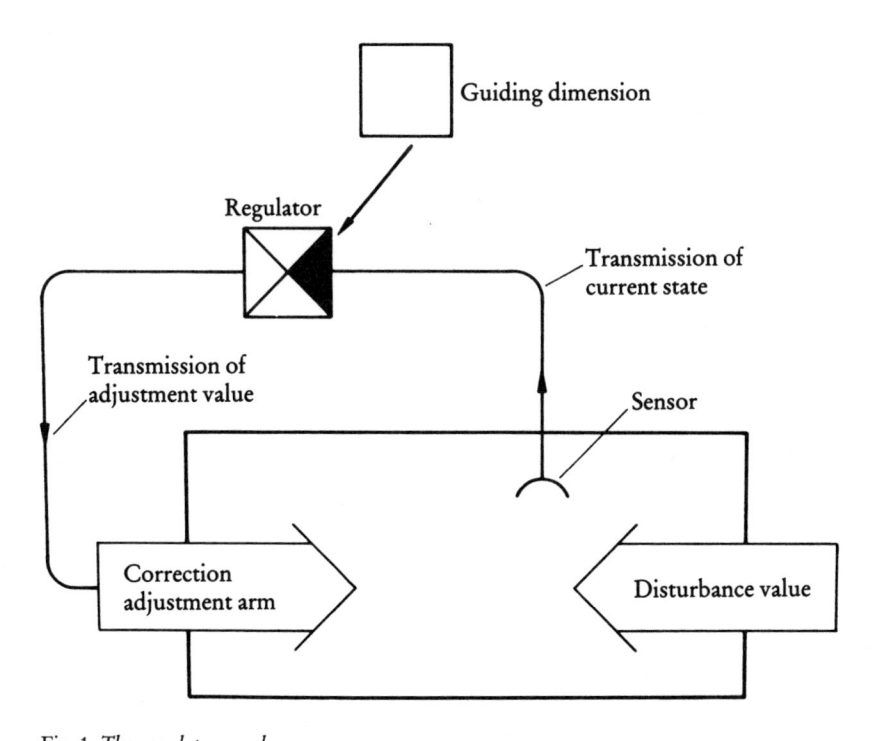

Fig. 1: *The regulatory cycle*
In the sensor, the nominal value is compared with the actual value in the regulatory pathway established by the sensor. Where there are differences that exceed the tolerance boundary of the system, the regulator gives the adjustment arm an appropriate adjustment value (correction), and the resulting action of the adjustment arm brings about the correction in the substrate.

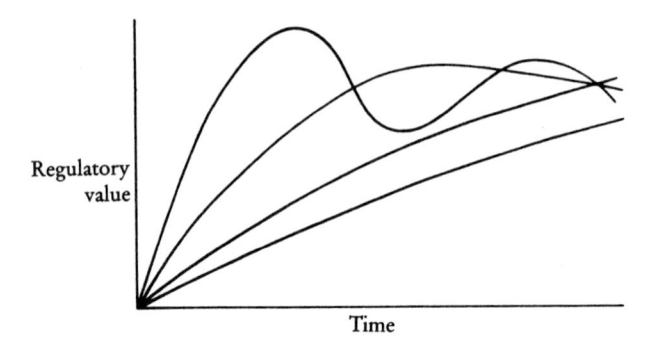

IMMEDIATE RESPONSE OF A SYSTEM, depending on the REGULATORY QUALITY

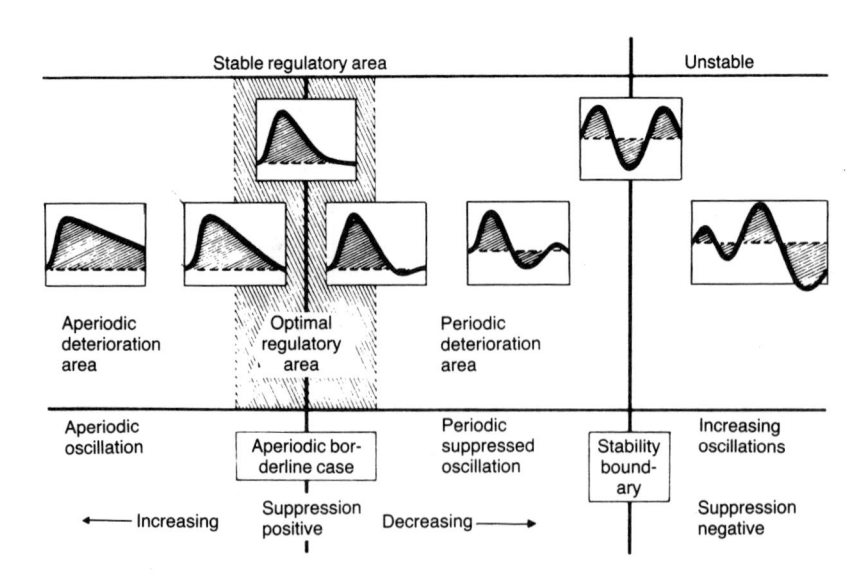

Stable regulatory area			Unstable
Aperiodic deterioration area	Optimal regulatory area	Periodic deterioration area	
Aperiodic oscillation	Aperiodic borderline case	Periodic suppressed oscillation	Stability boundary	Increasing oscillations
←—— Increasing	Suppression positive	Decreasing ——→		Suppression negative

Fig. 2: *Oscillatory behaviour*
Above: immediate response with adjustment of normal value. Below: levelling-out and return with short-term stimuli (needle function).

Regulatory Quality and Its Disturbance

The function of a regulatory cycle (system) is characterized by its regulatory quality and can be determined by observation of the conformation of one or several parameters. Here, the conformation behaviour is defined as the change from one steady state of the system to another steady state.

Optimal regulatory quality accords dampened oscillatory behaviour, where the regulatory aim is reached in the shortest time, with the minimal energy loss, which conforms to the principle of economy.

Periodically denatured-labile oscillatory types of behaviour are the pathological types of regulation, where the regulatory aim is exceeded primarily through rapid and excessive oversteer, and is only reached finally after several after-oscillations. The *resonance reaction* is a special type of periodic disturbance, where the after-oscillations become higher and higher, the compensatory value is exceeded and the entire system breaks down in a *tipping* reaction. The second dysreglatory possibility is *aperiodic-inert* disturbance, where the regulatory aim is delayed or is not reached. Time and energy are lost through both types of disturbances – they do not correspond to the principle of economy, and since it is a primary task of regulation to maintain the vital functions in an optimal field, a pathological border area is reached.

Here, a situation that is mainly forgotten in practice has to be mentioned: even in the resting organism there are no fixed parameter adjustments; instead, all the values oscillate around a mean value, so that from the point of view of regulation there is no difference between "stable" functions and those that are recognized from their rhythmic changes.

The main causes of regulatory disturbance are:
1. System defects, and not only diseases of the regulatory pathway belong to these. Deficits in mediators, hormones, enzymes, etc., as well as of substances that are involved in their formation, have to be taken into consideration here. Electrolyte blockage due to pathological stress from heavy metals, as described by Perger also belong here. The consequence of these deficits is mainly aperiodic deterioration.
2. On the other hand, preloading of the regulatory system due to foreign energy leads to *oversteering*, which leads to lability of the oscillations. Here, it is not so much a matter of the strength of the foreign energy – particularly from the aspect of chronic diseases – as the duration of

effect of this energy. The typical example is a focal process with regulatory disturbances due to the focus, which correspond to the exhaustion phase within the *adaptation syndrome (Selye)*.

3. In this connection, the role of the intermeshing of the regulatory system in response to stimuli has to be mentioned, which mainly comes to light in the evaluation of regulatory tests: a disturbing factor (of pathogenic nature, or a test stimulus) that is fed into the system can, depending on the actual function at a variety of exits (measured substrates), bring about completely different oscillatory processes. In this way, in the presence of dysregulation, a test can show aperiodic deterioration with observation of the electrolytes, while the observation of oscillations of the vascular wall or the leukocyte reaction can show periodically-disturbed, labile behaviour.

In every case, deterioration of the oscillatory processes disturbs the two teleological basic principles of biocybernetics – *homeostasis* and *economy*. The organism works totally or partly uneconomically, which leads to it reaching its performance limit earlier. The simultaneously existing metabolic disturbances favour degenerative changes in those organs that, on the one side, have regulatory disturbance, and, for whatever other reason, are required to produce an increased work performance.

From the clinical-pathological point of view, a differentiation has to be made between the *stimulus-reaction model* in short-term stimuli (needle function) and the *adaptation model* in long-term stimuli. In the latter, there is an initial stage of minus values, which leads to the observed parameters lying above the normal level. In the later phases there is exhaustion of the regulatory capacity with reduction of the values and sinking of reactivity in the sense of *Selye's* adaptation syndrome. Here, many of the states termed "focal disease" can be be given a regulatory-pathological classification.

These spotlights on biocybernetic facts and principles only have the task of showing that the syndrome thinking of clinical medicine, which is fully justified in the acute field, has to lead to confusion in chronic *diseases* and *illnesses*. In these states, only *thinking in network relationships*, expanded by knowledge of the *regulatory* and *control systems*, as well as their hierarchical relationships, can bring positive results (literature on biocybernetics in *Keidel* 1979, *Drischel* 1973, *Hildebrandt* 1982).

Chronicity as a Biocybernetic Problem

Demonstration of the clinical dependence of chronic states on regulatory processes and their disturbance is given in the following results and observations from investigations from rehabilitation medicine. Here, the question of reproducability can be answered extensively, namely that this is related to regulation and dysregulation and their correction, and that the regulatory therapy procedure naturally has to be individually different, since the regulatory disturbance can be set off by a variety of factors in each patient.

Observations in Chronic Pulmonary Tuberculosis

Although tuberculosis no longer plays the important role it had 20–30 years ago when these investigations were carried out, they remain suitable for demonstrating typical pathogenetic and therapeutic patterns within the framework of chronicity. However, it should not be forgotten that there is no question of the etiology of the tuberculous infection – the problem dealt with is *deterioration* into *chronicity*, and it also has to be noted that in spite of the intermittently epidemic character of tuberculosis, the mycobacterium tuberculosis is a microorganism with low human pathogenicity.

Pathogenetic Investigations

For an explanation of the extent to which the clinical manifestations of tuberculosis are dependent on secondary factors, 1542 case histories were evaluated from the following points of view.
1. Was there a unilateral stress before the first manifestation of the lung process (trauma, operation, organic disease, etc.)?
2. Was the start of the tuberculosis predominantly unilateral (ignoring minimal contralateral foci)?
3. To what extent is there agreement between the prestressed side and the side where tuberculosis began?

Result: 503 of 1542 patients fulfilled criteria 1 and 2; of these 75.5% developed the disease on the same side as the prestress.

In 145 patients, undoubted, objective, unilateral previous findings were documented, in agreement with the case history information. In this group the agreement between the prestressed side and the side of development was 93.8% (*Bergsmann* 1963).

This investigation shows clearly that apart from the biochemical cascade, of whose reality there can be no doubt, definite control processes play a role in the pathogenesis of chronic diseases, and this will be discussed in more detail later.

Therapeutic Results

Starting from the investigations described above, we attempted to influence the process with therapeutic methods that have regulatory activity. Neural therapy and acupuncture seemed to be suitable. First of all, it must be pointed out that the only patients included in these investigations were those whose sputum was permanently converted by several months of optimal chemo-antibiotic therapy, but who still had, as before, residual cavities. The last-used triple combination of tuberculostatics was retained in all patients.

After 3–5 months of regular regulatory therapy the cavities disappeared in every case.

6 months were needed for a giant cavity that had been documented as resistant to therapy for 6 years.

With neural therapy, extrapulmonary foci were loaded with local anesthetic in the sense of stoerfeld (disturbance field) therapy, and at the same time thoracic projection zones of the pulmonary process were infiltrated. Acupuncture therapy consisted of a variety of programs that are effective on the lungs, each adjusted to the individual situation.

Breakdown of Hyperergic Reactions

This detail is given special description due to its general validity, although we only had our first experience and knowledge in the field of tuberculosis (*Bergsmann* 1968). After we had learned that patients with hyperactive tuberculosis and high tuberculin skin sensitivity were inevitably subject to secondary disturbances (foci-disturbance fields), the confirmed foci in a group of patients with high tuberculin sensitivity were surrounded regularly with local anesthetic before starting chemo-antibiotic therapy. The result was a reduction in sensitivity by a factor of about 1000.

The fact of *tuberculin allergy did not change, but the allergometric* degree regressed.

Analogous therapeutic results could also be achieved in focus-caused *hyper-reactivity* of the bronchial mucosa, a finding that is frequently evaluated as incipient bronchial asthma.

Increase in General Performance Capacity

In the initial phase of rehabilitation after prolonged severe diseases, the adynamism and lack of drive of the patients often hinders the necessary training. A trial with therapy methods that are effective on regulation can be a great help here.

After we had seen in individual observations that acupuncture and disturbance field (foci, stoerfeld) anesthesia can have a good effect, we examined the effect of these methods on groups of 20 rehabilitation patients aged between 18 and 40 years, using ergometry.

The acupuncture group was treated with a program suggested by *Bischko*, and the neural therapy group was treated individually by switching-off established disturbance fields by using local anesthesia.

Prior to and 24 hours after a single treatment, the performance capacity of the patients was tested using pulse-regulated ergometry. *Method:* the ergometer brake was regulated from the pulse rate of the patient; we had laid down a working pulse of 120/min for reasons of industrial law. The actual performance was recorded continually over 10 minutes pedalling work. Both the initial performance peak and the total performance over 10 minutes were increased with statistical significance by both forms of treatment. Paralle blood gas and spirometric tests also showed that the oxygen uptake capacity was also increased after the therapy.

For this reason, both treatment methods were adopted in the therapy routine of the rehabilitation center. Later, we were able to investigate and judge positively other regulatory therapy methods, using the same systems.

Treatment of Tension Pain Syndromes by Neural Therapy

In order to check the effects of focus disturbance field anesthesia in a larger number of patients, the clinically established foci were loaded with local anesthetic after completion of the admission examination and before carrying out any other form of therapy; this was carried out in the Gröbming rehabilitation center, with the agreement of the patients. After 24 hours the patients were questioned about the effects, and the answers were noted in the case histories according to a +3 to –2 code. A series of case histories were selected at random from the archives, and evaluated.

Number of patients	518	= 100%
after 24 hours		
Complaint-free or minimal residual complaints.	113	= 22%
Significant improvement	156	= 30%
Total positive results	269	= 52%

Although the title "pain therapy" might attract spectacular casuistics, these figures should only speak for the method, without comment. However, it has to be emphasized that *no topical pain technique with therapeutic local anesthesia was used, and that the treatment result was only achieved by neural therapeutic* breakdown *of the existing* dysregulation.

However, consequent use of focus and disturbance field treatment within the framework of in-patient pain and function therapy also brought about an *economic* effect, due to a drastic reduction in the costs of analgesics, antirheumatics and corticoids, which is comparable to the "cost sparing" effect of focal stabilization published by *Perger*.

Regulatory Therapy for Respiration and Circulation

Successful regulatory therapy is marked by a reduction of connective tissue turgor and muscle tone, with a change in respiratory movement. If a false stereotype of respiratory movement existed before starting treatment, surrounding a disturbance field with local anesthetis brings about a change of respiration to the normal pattern.

Normal respiration is marked by optimal flank expansion as a result of the cooperation of the "bucket handle movement" of the first ribs (action of the scalenus) with the expansive movements of the lower ribs (second phase of diaphragmatic action) and the movement of the sternum, where the manubrium is retained at the same level in inspiration and expiration.

In contrast to this, in *false* respiration, the sternum remains elevated in inspiration, and the "bucket handle movement" becomes more difficult, or ceases, and part of the flank expansion caused by the diaphragm is lost. Since, apart from this, part of the insertion of the diaphragm is carried towards the dome due to the inspiratory elevation of the thorax, the first part of the action of the diaphragm is lost to the respiratory process (*Bergsmann* and *Eder* 1982).

In unilateral stress to the organism, for example in unilateral foci or unilateral disturbance of the function of the axial organ, this false respiration can only appear on the affected side, while the unaffected side acts normally. There is then *asymmetry* and *asynchronism* of the respiratory movement.

In otherwise undisturbed pulmonary and thoracic function, the volume and capacity of the lungs is not altered by false movement, or it is only altered slightly. However, the result is a significant hindrance to respiratory work, and significantly more work is needed for the same ventilatory action, with correspondingly more use of oxygen. The result is that dyspnea appears with relatively low stress stages, as compared with normal respiration. The result is however also that the patient stressed in this way automatically strives to live with significantly less respiratory work – he is *hypodynamic*. The inspiratory thoracic movement is, however, not only active in respiration, apart from the peripheral muscle pump it is the strongest centrally-directed power for the circulatory low pressure system. Its disturbance has equally limiting effects on the lungs and the circulation, and since cardiac systole is also strengthened by the expiratory pressure increase, cardiac performance is also adversely affected by false respiration.

Circulatory analysis studies using *Schellong's* orthostasis test show that in unilateral stress and corresponding unilateral respiratory asymmetry on the side of the stress, there is a significant reduction in blood pressure amplitude in the standing period of the test.

However, respiratory movement does not only have an effect on ventilation and circulation; in the end, all organs are under the influece of rhythmic respiratory pressure variations. On the other hand, the functional state of the viscera also affects the tone and phasic action of the chest and abdominal musculature via the segmental reflex system, so that one can refer to a *mechano-visceral interaction*, with respiratory movement as its central point.

As our investigations have shown (*Bergsmann* 1986), these interconnections do not only have great significance in lung diseases; in patients

Schellong I Simultaneous bilateral

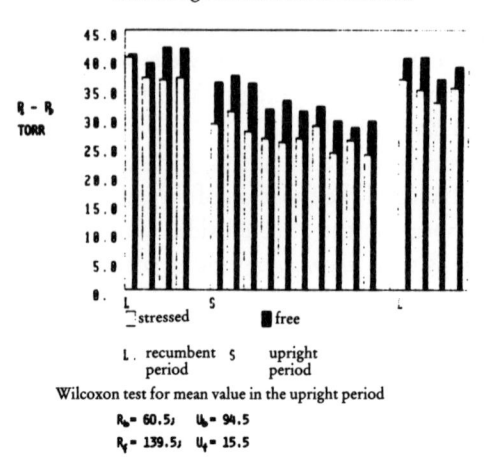

R - R
TORR

L stressed   S   ■ free   L

L . recumbent S upright
  period   period
Wilcoxon test for mean value in the upright period
R_s = 60.5; U_s = 94.5
R_f = 139.5; U_f = 15.5

Fig. 3: Schellong I-Test Bilateral-Simultaneous
With the simultaneous-bilateral orthostasis test, the blood pressure amplitude on the side with less respiratory excursion or false respiration is less than that on the side with normal inspiratory movements.

with functional disturbances due to the vertebra outside the thoracic spine we have also seen false stereotypes of respiratory movement in 68.3% of those investigated, and in 57% of the clinically healthy. As a result of the multiple regulatory disturbances caused by this, and the penalties for general performance capacity, this complex can be classified in the field of the *risk factors* for the occurrence of multiform degenerative illnesses.

The Pathogenetic Consequences

The empirical observations described in the previous chapter, and clinical-experimental results, can be expanded and extended any number of times. However, with the sciences of normal and pathological *physiology*, expanded by the science of the ground system according to *Pischinger* and *Heine*, they result in a clear picture of the pathogenesis of chronic diseases. However, the difference between *etiology* (the science of cause) and *pathogenesis* (the origins and development of a disease) has to be emphasized, because the various etiological factors in clinical science are not brought into question. However, the *"chronicity"* factor belongs to the field of pathogenesis!

The "Tip of the Iceberg"

In this connection, chronic diseases can be compared with an iceberg; for the base – namely the underlying causes – is hidden. The patient seeks out the doctor due to foreground complaints, mainly due to general or particular infirmity, to general discomfort and/or stress symptoms, or to pain symptoms. The primary complaints are the tip of the iceberg.

The Sensory-Motor Control System

In the end, almost every primary complaint symptom is of a sensory-motor nature. For this reason, the reader should be reminded briefly of the most important sensory-motor control and processing systems, without going into every detail.

1. The Segmental-Regulatory Complex

This is the most peripheral switching system, through which all the formations attached to a spinal segment are in functional relationship.

The control is accompanied by the fact that where there is disease of an internal organ, the function of autonomically controlled pathways on the body surface, such as muscle tone, sweat secretion, etc., is altered, but that the function of the internal organ can also be altered by therapeutic measures on the body surface, as is confirmed by the efficacy of the application of heat and poultices, as well as neural therapy and other medical regulatory treatments.

The autonomic nervous system is connected to the spinal segments between T2 (facultative T 1) and L 2 (facultative T 3). It is true that it has not yet been possible to confirm this in anatomical preparations, which would be impossible in view of the intermeshing of the peripheral ganglia

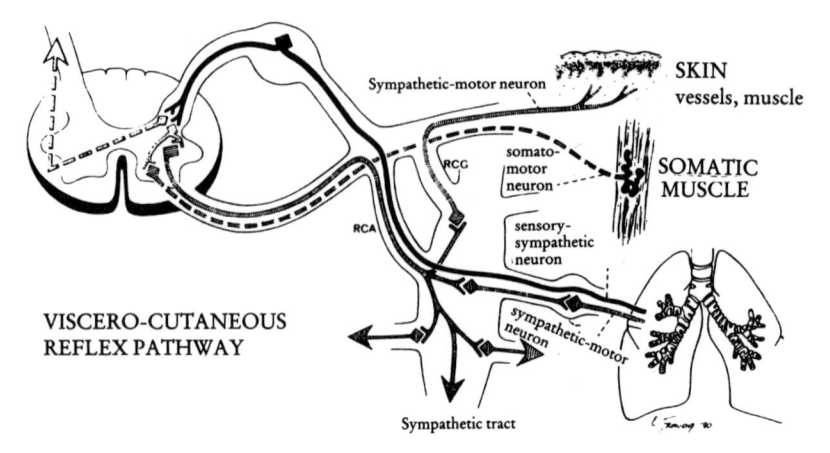

Fig. 4: The segmental regulatory complex
The functional intermeshing of all the substrates connected with the spinal segment is shown, with the viscerocutaneous reflex pathway as an example. Since not only the internal organ can alter the functions, but also the skin, muscle, etc., the term reflex is misguiding. This is a functional network

and plexuses, even in the future, but it has been possible to demonstrate the segmental arrangement of the autonomic nervous system experimentally.

The sensory supply of the skin is provided by dendritic branching of the nerve endings, so that every nerve supplies a *"receptive field"*. At the borders of the dermatomes there are sites of greater sensitivity due to the multiple overlappings of the nerve supply, and these mainly correspond to acupuncture points, according to *Melzack* (1973).

Information from the periphery is altered into signals by the nerve endings or other sensors, and these signals are transmitted to the control cells of the posterior horn. Physiologists and clinicians have discussed a system of gate control for a long time. Here, *Melzack* offers a model for thought, which offers sufficient explanatory possibilites for most clinical and therapeutic problems:

A control cell is sited before the synapse with the transmitter cell, and this feeds back the afferent fibers presynaptically. The control cell is inhibited by signals in thin fibers (mainly autonomic) and stimulated by signals in thick fibers (mainly somatic). Stimulation means throttling back the information input and inhibition of an unlimited inflow of information.

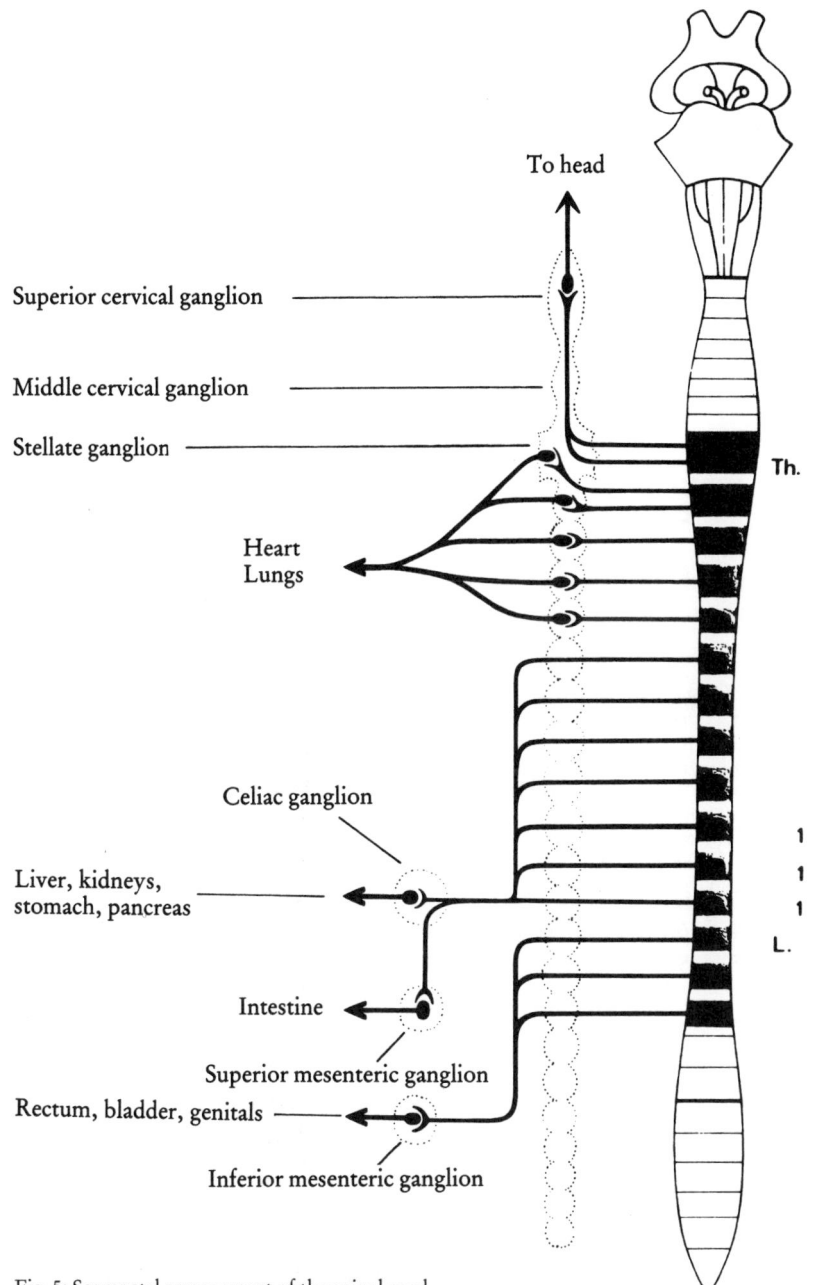

Fig. 5: Segmental arrangement of the spinal cord.
The segmental-regulatory complex is repeated in each spinal segment; from T2 to L2 (facultatively from T1 to L3) the sympathetic tract is also connected in tiers.

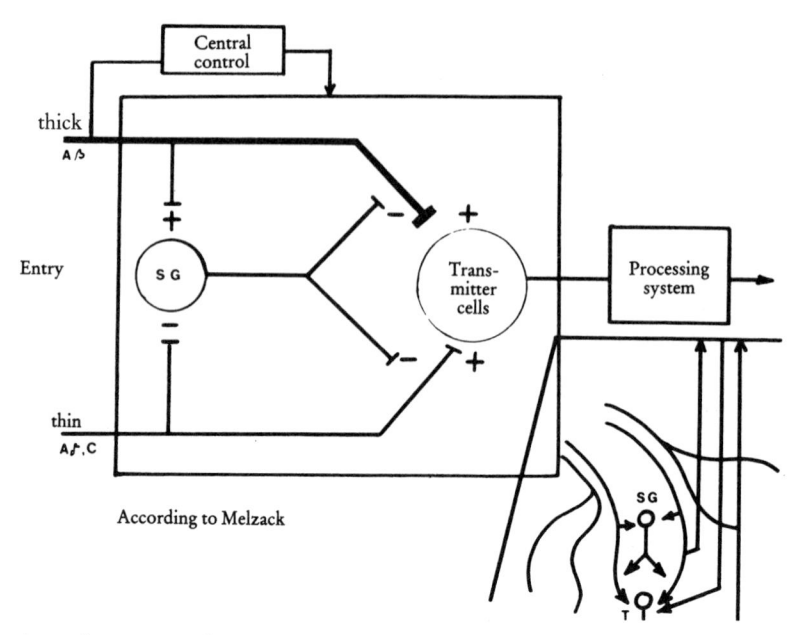

Fig. 6: *The gate control system*
Posterior horn entry control is generally recognized, but the details are still under discussion. The system postulated by *Melzack* and *Wall* is suitable as a basis for thought in describing the projection processes and mechanism of types of therapy that have regulatory effectiveness. The posterior horn entry has thick and thin fibers. A controll cell is connected in series with the posterior horn transmitter cells (SG); they have presynaptic feedback with the afferent fibers. The control cells are inhibited by afferent signals in thin fibers, and stimulated by the signals in thick fibers.
The result is: the more information that arrives via thin fibers, the less inhibited is the flow of signals in the spinal cord. Through this it can be stimulated over the pain threshold. The more information from thick, somatic fibers, the more the control cell is stimulated and the posterior horn entry suppressed.

Since a signal-flooding of the posterior horn occurs with disinhibition of input, the sum of the afferents exceedes the pain threshold. On the other hand, when the posterior horn is throttled back, the quantity of information sinks below the pain threshold. Acupuncture with actuation of the somatic afferents (thick fibers) and neural therapy with switching off the afferents via thin fibers are thus both suitable for closing the gate control system, and thus reducing pain. Control of the gate control system can also be used to interpret the working of other forms of regulatory therapy.

Naturally, the gate control system is under central control, and equally naturally, the information is transmitted and processed via the vertical hierarchy of the central nervous formations and programs.

2. Regulatory Control of the Musculature

Like all other organs, the musculature is included in the segmental-regulatory complex. The regulatory response to functional or pathogenic information consists of changes in tone which are regulated by the gammamotoric-tonic system, where the primary response to a stimulus is mostly an increase in tone.

Muscle tone is mainly varied by three centers:
1. The cerebellum, where, in particular, the centers for balance and statics lie – a second balance center is presumed to exist in the cervical part of the spine.
2. The centers of the formatio reticularis, where, due to the close relationship to the superior autonomic centers, muscle tone is adjusted to the vital autonomic functions.
3. The segmental reflex complexes, where the local muscle tone is adjusted to the general segmental function.

In order to be able to carry out coordinated *complex movements,* programs are opened up in the interneuron pool of the spinal cord during postempbryonic development, as well as in the higher centers. This takes place in every learning process – from erect walking, speaking and writing, to handwork and sports training. The result of these programs is that no individual muscle can be activitated alone, but only the complete *kinetic chain*. Differentiation of complex movements, as regards their extent, strength, etc., takes place via spinal-segmental inhibitory mechanisms.

The tone system is also included in this kinetic control. The result is that in segmentally-stimulated muscle tone, the muscles connected to the segmental-regulatory complex are primarily those that are hypertonic. However, since they are part of a kinetic chain, the hypertonic state passes over to the entire chain. The result is a tone situation that oversteps the segment, corresponding to the course of the kinetic chain. These chain symptoms have clinical diagnostic significance as (continue on page 101):

Supraspinal centers

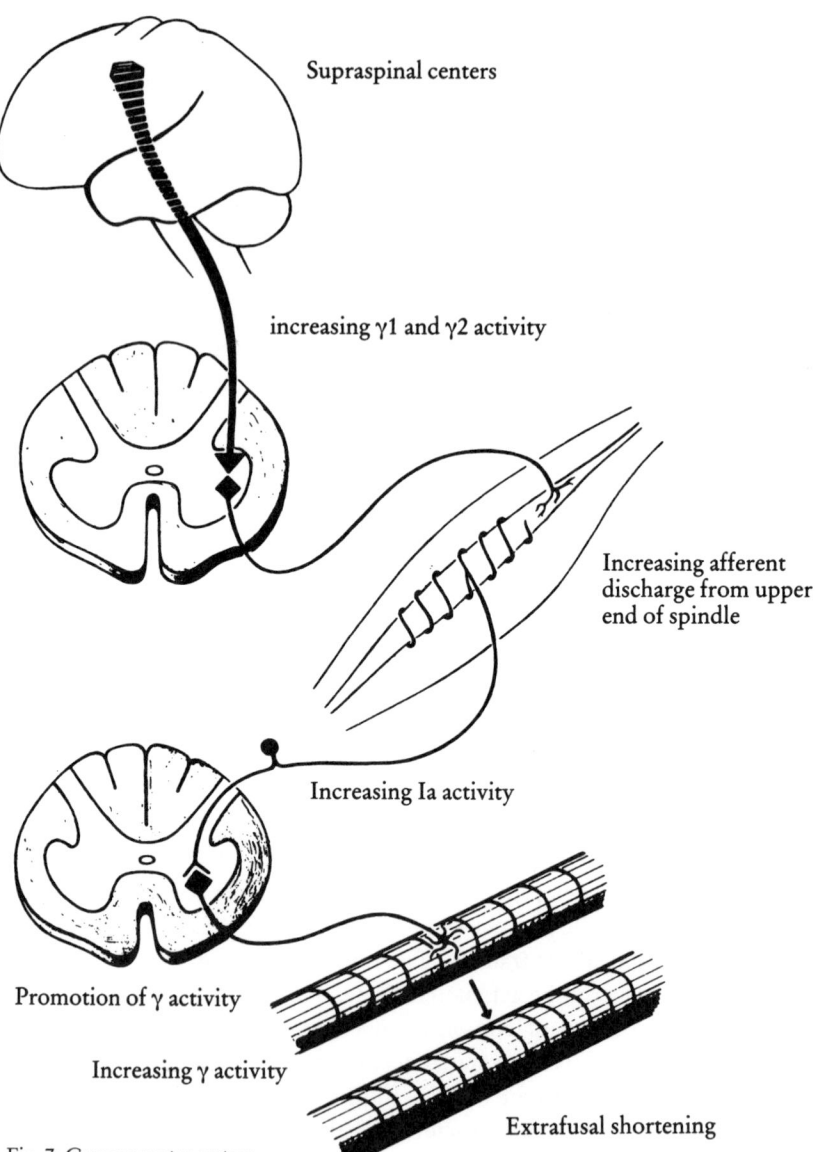

increasing γ1 and γ2 activity

Increasing afferent discharge from upper end of spindle

Increasing Ia activity

Promotion of γ activity

Increasing γ activity

Extrafusal shortening

Fig. 7: *Gamma motor system*
As the second neural system of the musculature, the gamma motor system has autonomous responsibility for spatial attitude and position (antigravitation) and muscle tone. It also acts as a servosystem for the alpha motor system. Central control takes place via the cerebellum (antigravitation) and the formatio reticularis (intermeshing and adjustment with autonomic functions). As stretch-feelers, the muscle spindles are responsible for regulation of local tension, but their sensitivity is controlled by the centers.

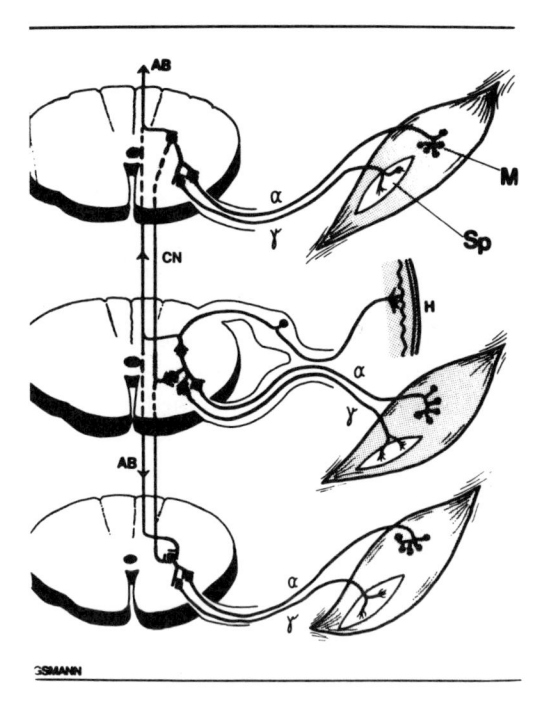

Fig. 8: *Trans-segmental muscle circuits*
Movement complexes have to be able to be carried out with automatic preprogramming. On the one hand, the basis of these programs is the innervation of the muscles involved in the same spinal segment, but for the most part it lies in the postembryonic circuits in the interneuron pools of the spinal cord and midbrain. Programming takes place in every motor learning process.

1. due to them, the change in function brought about by segmental-regulatory action obscures the symptoms beyond the segment,
2. but by following the symptoms from peripherally to proximally, e.g. by palpation, the symptom chain leads to the initiator,
3. through this, with peripheral therapy, a long-range effect on the initiator can be achieved,
4. and these radiating tonic-algetic symptoms are by far the most frequent symptoms in daily medical practice.

A further aspect is the parallel between these tension symptoms and the musculo-tendinous meridians of acupuncture.

3. The Muscular Maximal Point System

Reflex muscular hypertonicity can exceed the pain threshold to a degree that varies from individual to individual, but even in minimal, pain-free tensions, maximal points (triggers, etc.) can be found in every muscle, with stereotyped localization; with gentle finger pressure, they present as shallow skin depressions with a smooth surface. With stronger pressure, hardenings of various sizes can be felt in tense muscle; the pressure sets off a pain sensation, as well as pain radiating into a reference zone lying in the course of the kinetic chain to which this muscle belongs.

Here, only the importance of these maximal points for diagnosis and therapy can be mentioned; systematics and further details can be read in *Brugger* (1980), *Travell* and *Simons* (1983), and *Bergsmann* and *Bergsmann* (1988). According to our own observations (*Bergsmann* 1983), good acupuncture points always correspond to maximal points.

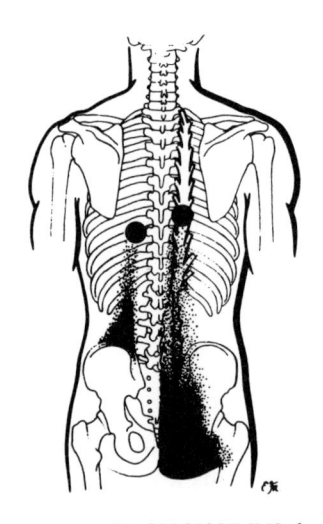

MUSCULUS LONGISSIMUS thoracis

Fig. 9: *Tension symptom example*
Like the alphamotor movement innervation, reflex muscular nociceptive hypertonicity follows the course of the kinetic chains. Trans-segmental pain symptoms (pseudoradicular) arise through this. Maximal points lie in the tensed muscle, with stereotyped localization.
Circle = maximal point
Black surface = the muscles referred pain

Knowledge of this system is an essential precondition for functional diagnosis of the movement system, and for regulatory therapy.

Diagnostically, there is practically nothing better than the palpating finger, even though these points are also marked by changes in the skin potential, electrical resistance and conductivity, as well as changes in infrared radiation.

4. The Role of the Axial Organ in Regulation

It is mostly forgotten that the spine is not only the center of positional and movement mechanism, but has many connections with the pathogenesis of regulatory disturbances and degenerative diseases, since each stimulus set off by the segmental-regulatory system leads to metabolic impairment and thus favours degenerative changes. On the other hand, the simultaneously raised muscle tone (mostly unilateral) means mechanical stress to the axial organ with lasting disturbances of statics and dynamics and the development of functional disturbances in the movement segments. Degenerations and disturbances of function are secondary sources of patho-infomation; they feed back into the segmental-regulatory complex and can thus lead to self-perpetuation of the regulatory disturbance. In addition, participation by the spine can lead to a primary, unilateral, disturbance of function on the contralateral side, if additional contralateral dysfunctions appear in tendons, fascia and joints during rotation processes. The central significance of the axial organ is that the movement segments are vulnerable from practically everywhere, but that they themselves can adversely affect practically all the functions of the organism.

5. Spinal Afference and Subordinate Control Systems

This is not the place to yet again repeat the anatomy of the cerebral pathways and the higher centers, but the impression should not be given that only the segmental-regulatory complexes participate in pathogenesis, symptoms and therapy. The information is passed to the higher centers via the known centripetal pathways, and processed there according to function.

After the segmental-regulatory complex, the rhombo-spinal control system is the most important center for the formation of segmental reflexes. The various segmental-regulatory functions are controlled there, and the visceromotor as well as the somatomotor reflexes are both set in motion and controlled.

The formatio reticularis lies in the rhombo-mesencephalic control system. Its main task is stabilization of the internal milieu and in the intimate relationship between the autonomic centers and the gamma motor system. The result is that this area is responsible for the coordination of autonomic and somatic functions.

The hypothalamus, the diencephalon-hypothalamic control system, also takes part in the coordination of autonomic and somatic functions, since it has a key position in the defence of internal and external stressors, and also participates in the triggering of behaviour patterns and moods.

In the limbic system, all afferent signals are processed to complexes, and are coordinated with the environment in feedback with the information from the hypothalamus.

All external factors are processed in the neocortical system, and coordinated with the information from the autonomic and somatic centers. Discussing the specific cortical functions, such as consciousness, mentality, etc., would exceed the parameters of this part of the book.

The "Base of the Iceberg"

The Ground System

The clinical picture that is primarily accessible to the medical practitioner is based on histochemical and biochemical disturbances of function, whose point of initiation is function and dysfunction of the *ground system*, which is discussed in this book; it is therefore not necessary to go into structure and function further in this part. However, to understand the leading role of the function of the ground system in the pathogenesis of chronic diseases and degenerative diseases, it has to be emphasized that the ground system is not only the starter for information at cells, the humoral system and the nervous system, but that the function of the system itself can be altered by every functional disturbance of the tissues. This is essential, particularly with regard to multiple feedback mechanisms, without which chronicity and degeneration are not easily understood.

The time factor plays a significant role in this connection. Without it, the effects of long-lasting minimal stresses (foci, disturbance fields) can not be explained or understood.

Every short-lasting stimulus leads primarily to partial depolarization of proteoglycans, which is eliminated at once in open and functionally capable systems through charge replacement. Minimal duration stimuli from localized inflammatory foci are thus the cause of lasting depolarization processes, which eventually have to lead to structural changes in the entire ground system; at the end of this degeneration process, the transformation is in the direction of a gel. This means that there is an alteration in the direction of biological inactivity, as in every other colloid that loses its surface charge.

At the moment there are no experimental results that lead to a direct or analogous conclusion concerning the effect of the stimulus on the semi-crystalline water fields lying between the molecular filaments, but it can be assumed that they also alter or lose their polarization, structure and order, as a result of the charge alteration in the environment, and through this, a further ground system organization factor disappears. In this connection, attention has to be drawn to the investigations carried out by *Trincher* (cit. from *Heine*), who established that the proportion of crystalline water decreases with warming, and according to whose opinion life itself is not possible without crystalline water.

The cell, whose metabolism and biological activity is regulated by the ground system, according to *Pischinger* and *Heine,* is, however, a generator of electromagnetic information. According to calculations made by *Fröhlich* (1980), with a membrane thickness of 0.0000006 cm and a potential difference of 0.1 V, a field strength of 100,000 V/cm can be expected. These high, unstable field strengths cause oscillation in membranes and their dipoles. According to *Fröhlich,* the result from the relationship between the speed of sound and membrane thickness is a resonating oscillation in the microwave field (about 1 TeraHz).

More recent research by *Popp* (1983) and *Klima* (1981, 1987), showed that the electromagnetic oscillations of coherent light present an information system for all living organisms, which had previously been given little attention, where the transition of oxygen from the stimulated single state to the molecular triple state was recognized as a laser source with a wavelength of 634 nm. This system appears to be highly significant in the field of cell regeneration, but from personal laser investigations (*Bergsmann*

1983), it is also capable of releasing resonance and damping phenomena in low frequencies (ELF).

Transmission of Information

It seems to be certain that these changes have their primary effect on the immediate environment as a result of the electrolability and coherence of the ground system, and that they only affect the entire organism when they are of long duration, thus altering regulatory quality. In addition, every denatured regulatory process creates the preconditions for further worsening of the regulatory basis, and it is also necessary to point out that not only neural regulatory processes, but also local tissue and humoral regulatory systems are affected, and that the interaction of a variety of regulatory systems is affected by this, in the sense of the macroorganic network.

The spreading of the dysfunction of the ground system certainly does not take place suddenly, but with feedback with neural and humoral systems. Here, a pattern might be taken from the clinical terminology of compartments. This is justified to the extent that limits are set to the information spread by charge displacements due to the isolation properties of serous membranes, septa and fascia; however, according to *Nordenström* (1983) these can be crossed by building up biological connections via lymphatics, arteries and veins, in the sense of biologically closed electric circuits (BCEC).

However, the electrolability and oscillation capacity of the ground system structures also requires their sensitivity to electrostatic and electromagnetic environmental influences, such as static fields, air electricity charges and electromagnetic impulse fields, the so-called spherics. This is all the more so, as *Heine* was able to demonstrate, since the ground system is stretched out from below against the surface of the body in the form of cylinders that surround the superficial fascia perforating nervous and vascular bundles. Since this "Heine cylinder" is invested in a membrane like structure that has little conductivity, we are dealing with an organ that can do more than take up and process mechanical qualities. In the sense of electromagnetism, it is also capable of oscillation, and it can even be expected that it can be identified as the organ of perception for electromagnetic and magnetic dimensions. With this, a further bridge would be built regarding the understanding of weather sensitivity and the effects of prolonged minimal electric and magnetic stresses.

On the other hand, the existence of the Heine cylinders also provides the explanation of the fact that organic regulatory processes can be altered effectively by a variety of completely different techniques, such as massage, magnetic fields, ELF electric fields, needle pricks, local anesthesia and laser beams that can be inserted into the organism via acupuncture points and alterning persistantly the organic regulation processes.

The system of pyrhoelectrical and piezoelectrical chains discovered by *Athenstaedt* (1977) also has to be mentioned in this connection. According to this author, the entire organism is interwoven with chains of piezoelectrical dipolar molecules with their polarity acting in the same direction. The structural proteoglycans belong to these piezoelectrical chain systems; their individual molecules are dipoles, and they are capable of oscillation due to their spiral structure. In addition, their molecular structure is varied by the fibroblasts in dysfunction of the proteoglycans of the ground system. This provides a further reason for degenerative processes in the movement system, and it is clear that these pathological variants have oscillation and resonance properties that differ from those of normal glycoproteins.

On the other hand, dipolar molecules not acting in the same direction can be made to act in the same direction by relatively weak external and internal fields, and therefore form electrets, which have the same properties as the primary piezoelectrical chains. In addition to this, *Athenstaedt* established – in dried preparations – that the positive poles of the piezoelectrical chains always point in the direction of growth. However, the piezoelectrical function of the structural glycoproteins seems to have special importance for the basic information system of the organism: piezoelectrical properties require that on the one hand electrical fields occur with pressure changes, and on the other that electromagnetic fields of a certain resonance frequency are altered to mechanical oscillations. The latter lead to strong periodic pressure changes in the surroundings, which can not be without effects on the metabolic stream through the molecular sieve of the extracellular matrix and on the structure of the water region. We were able to produce evidence of the modulatory effect of laser frequencies on the frequency of muscular activity (*Bergsmann* 1983).

With this large number of information systems, consideration always has to be given to the fact that there is an uninterrupted exchange of information between them, and that there are multiple functioning feedback possibilities in the network system. Up to now, the author is not aware of any diagnostic system that only addresses one of these systems alone.

In practice, evaluation of the state of function of the ground system with humoral parameters is difficult. Here, in accordance with the latest morphological knowledge, the point diagnosis system offers a way out. Details can be found in the chapter entitled "The Point – the Window to the Ground System" (p. 120).

Regulatory Disintegration

Regulatory disintegration has shown itself to be particularly fruitful as a general patho-cybernetic concept in both pathogenetic research and practical regulatory diagnosis, since it provides an explanation of regulatory diagnostic phenomena, processes in the development of disease, and tissue degeneration.

Initially there is regulatory disturbance, which affects the correponding dermatomes, myotomes, etc. through interaction with false segmental-regulatory control, and also alters vasomotion and other autonomic functions in the quadrants in question via the autonomic nervous system, to the extent that the entire metabolism and its regulatory processes – as well as the basic information systems – work differently in comparison to the undisturbed parts of the organism. The difference does not only affect the levels of the compared parameters, time displacements also occur. With increasing strength of the stimuli, and with the inclusion of regulatory processes, this primarily local phenomenon develops itself into a set of unilateral regulatory symptoms. This only results in a general disease at a relatively late stage, under the influence of secondary and tertiary factors.

Within the framework of *degenerative deterioration,* the disproportion between somatic musculotendinous tension states and disturbed vasomotion acquire the role of being the initiators of degeneration of the movement system, and here too, the disturbed ground system functions as the regulatory interface.

In this connection, it is impossible to deal with all the physiological details in a clinical paper. However, from the material available, functional disturbance of the ground system and the deterioration of all oscillatory processes resulting from this, as well as the disturbed interaction of the subsystems in the network of the macroorganism are the *base of the iceberg.*

Minimal, Chronic Lasting Stress (Focus, Disturbance Field, Stoerfeld)

The regulatory systems and their pathways summarized here are stressed and disturbed by factors of clinical disease pictures. Minimal, chronic inflammations, which can only be detected with difficulty and scientific precision due to their lack of local symptoms, feed information into them. This, as a result of the minimal extension and absence of activity of these processes, is mainly subliminal, and no symptoms are produced in the sense of a stimulus-reaction pattern. However, since they, although undetected, often give off this information for years or decades, they place all the regulatory systems (cellular, tissue, humoral and neural) under preliminary stress. The result is mostly periodic deterioration, namely lability of the oscillatory processes, with the result that there is an excessive response to all additional stimuli. In this way, common, non-pathogenic stimuli acquire pathological status.

Primarily, this lability concerns the segmental-regulatory complex to which the focus is connected. Since nutrition and clearance are also affected, degenerative metabolism occurs, which can be demonstrated in the movement system in particular, since degenerative metabolism combined with multiple movement processes creates a *locus minoris resistentiae* in this system. However, there are adverse metabolic effects on all other organs.

The further consequences are an extension of this regulatory change, and this leads to the appearance of regulatory disintegration. The crossing-over of the regulatory symptoms to the contralateral side shows, as already discussed, the secondary affection of the axial organ.

If this labilized system is affected by a secondary noxious stimulus, or a common stimulus, this *"secondary stress"* is answered inadequately and excessively, and sets off a *"remote disturbance"* (fernstoerung), whose localization is determined by the point where the secondary injury occured. Secondary injuries include all further stimuli, including secondary. A focal disease which is monofocal is extremely unusual.

However, the findings by *Selye* (1953) on the adaptation syndrome are also valid for minimal stress; according to these, with lasting stress (adaptation model), exhaustion with numbed reaction appears after a temporary tendency to overreaction.

Diagnostic Phenomena

Clinical regulatory diagnosis has to be carried out under three criteria:
1. *Localization diagnosis* to objectivize a local disturbance of function, which includes pain. Its use for detecting the initiating point of a disturbance of function is, however, much more important.
2. *Quality diagnosis* affects the deterioration of the oscillatory processes, or the answer to the question of which oscillatory process is deteriorated, and how much, since this can be decisive for therapy.
3. *Localization the cause of disturbance.* This is important from the point of view of beginning therapy, as causal therapy can only be initiated via localization of the initiator of a disturbance of function.

The *establishment of regulatory disintegration* is supported by localization diagnosis, as well as the actual functional disturbance and the starter. Mainly, the varying regulatory quality decides the differentiation between these two phenomena.

Diagnostic Guidelines

Both manual and technical methods follow the physiological guidelines, as already mentioned.

Colloid State

The colloid state of the cutis and subcutis determines the diagnosis, both by palpation and by electrical measurements, and since it depends on the perfusion of the capillaries, it can be set in analogy to the thermodiagnostic findings.

The swelling or shrinking of tissue colloid is regulated by autonomically controlled changes in the function of arteriovenous anastomoses (avA), and by the tone of the smooth muscles of the skin, which is varied by autonomic control. The avAs are rhythmically-working connections between the high pressure and low pressure systems of the circulation, and an anastomosis mainly consists of two to three vessels. In reflex stimulation of an area, primarily the precapillary and postcapillary sphincters increase their tone, which means that the final vascular network is not fully perfused. This leads, on the one hand, to hypoxia and acidosis of the tissue, with changes in the pH value and the fluid content of the colloid state of the tissue from "sol direction" to "gel direction". However, this alters the dielectrical constant of the tissue and thus all the bioelectrical functions and values. This also affects the radiation coefficient and local temperature. The second, mainly misunderstood effect of this process is that arterial shunt blood is mixed with venous blood, which means that all the blood constituents meant for use in the tissue (mainly oxygen) appear in increased amounts in the venous blood.

Projection Symptoms of Internal Organs

The formation of projection symptoms with the cooperation of the sensory-motor system has already been mentioned. It can be regarded as the primary cause of regulatory disintegration. The systemization of this "reflex sign of disease" was started by *Head* (1898) and *Mackenzie* (1911), and was summarized by *Hansen* and *Schliak* (1960). More recent investigations, particularly in the field of the movement system have, however, shown that the problem of organ projection greatly exceeds the symptoms in the skin and subcutaneous area, and that widely radiating symptom pictures can be formed with the inclusion of switching systems that cross over individual segments, but that these can be traced back to their origins through knowledge of the pathway system. These connections were presented recently by *Gleditsch* (1983) and *Bergsmann* and *Bergsmann* (1988).

Acupuncture and Meridians

The relationships between sensory-motor systems, kinetic chains and acupuncture points (*Bergsmann* and *Meng* 1982, *Bergsmann* and *Bergsmann* 1988) have already been mentioned above, as was the analogy between musculo-tendinous triggers and acupuncture points. The discovery of the "Heine cylinder" has brought yet another argument which helps the removal of the mystery of the acupuncture system. The empirically and experimentally confirmed functional diagnostic possibilities of this system could be discussed without any difficulty.

The equipment of the Heine cylinder with nerves and vessels appearing to have special significance in regards to functional diagnostic problems, since the electric and thermal functional difference from the surrounding skin can only be explained by this. The multiple possibilities of autonomic and somatic disturbances influencing the function of the point also find an explanation here.

As for ground system diagnosis and research, the acupuncture point can be regarded as the "window to the ground system" (see the appropriate section, p. 113).

Somatotopes

The somatotopes going beyond the basic projection and acupuncture system are only mentioned here, and will not be discussed further. *Gleditsch* (1983) gave an extensive description of the somatotopes.

Perfusion

Both central and peripheral perfusion factors such as flow volume and speed, and vascular bed parameters, are under direct or indirect autonomic influence, with the result that conclusions can be made on the autonomic status of the area investigated (see section on colloid).

Direct capillary microscopic investigation of the vascular bed can not be used in diagnosis due to time and cost factors, but investigations on the lip mucosa by *Brückle* (1963) are available. She established that stimuli alter the capillary flow in the vascular bed within the framework of regulatory stress. The changes range from flow acceleration to slowing of the flow, to flow reversal, to serum extravasation and the formation of paravascular "lakes". The analogy of these findings to the system of thought in *Ricker's Relation Pathology* (1924) cannot be ignored.

Humoral Parameters and Leukocytes

Observation of leukocytes and humoral parameters after standardized stimuli levels is one of the oldest functional diagnostic methods. The changes observed should be assessed by the biocybernetic criteria described above. As already mentioned, perfusion is subject to regulatory disintegration, and includes dysfunction of the arterio-venous anastomoses in the reflexly stressed quadrant in question, and asymmetrical humoral and cellular value can be observed in unilateral diseases.

Muscle Activity

Tonic initial stress of a kinetic chain requires that, in addition to work load, more muscular activity is required than in non-prestressed with the same load (*Bergsmann* 1988). From our own experience (*Bergsmann* 1983), myographic investigations are also suitable for understanding short-term rhythms under a variety of conditions, and to understand the problem of harmonic relationships objectively.

The Point: – the Window to the Ground System

Humoral regulatory diagnostic methods are mainly complex and time-intensive. This makes clinical ground system research significantly more difficult, and is certainly one reason for the fact that regulatory diagnosis can only carried through with delay, and that the methods that were already part of clinical diagnosis half a century ago were ignored.

Here, the discovery of the morphological structure of the acupuncture point and its relationship to the ground system opens up new possibilites, and the justification of already existing extraclinical diagnostic methods.

Morphology

A histological investigation by *Kellner* (1966) on 14,000 skin sections showed a more than chance accumulation of sensory elements at a variety of points (not all), but that there was no structural difference between a point and neutral skin.

Recently, *Heine* (1987) discovered that neurovascular bundles penetrate the superficial fascia in the points he investigated, and take a cylinder of extracellular matrix with them. This cylinder is closed-off by a layer of proteoglycans. It is also closed on its upper (external) side, although the nerve endings emerge there. The intensive contact of a relatively large and concentrated part of the extracellular matrix with the surface is a primary problem in ground system diagnosis. This makes technical measurement and interpretation possible.

Functional Possibilities of the Point Organ

According to *Heine's* description, this is a multifunctional organ:
- From the mechanical point of view it is a viscoelastic system consuming thrust and pressure.
- The proteoglycan network of the close to the surface lying organ is, in principle, capable of oscillation, and thus capable of reacting to electrical, electromagnetic and magnetic stimuli.
- A network of electrolabile molecular filaments provides a storage system for charges, namely an accumulator. However, due to its isolation capacity, the surrounding, impermeable layer gives more the impression of a condenser.
- As a result of their electrical lability, proteoglycans react to every quality of stimulus with depolarization and can transmit this in the ground system as a chain reaction. In this way the continuity of primary information mediation from the point to distant regions of the body is guaranteed.
- From the penetration of the ground system and the neurovascular bundle through the gap in the fascia, the possibility of muscle tension influencing the functional state of the point has to be considered, since every tension change alters the flow dynamics and the reactivity of the vascular bed.
- Finally, the vascular bundle is an indication of intensive connection with thermoregulation and the vasomotors.

This gives weighty indications for the diagnostic possibilities via point measurements, and it was necessary to investigate the question of the functional relationships between organ and point.

The Question of Functional Relationships

Decisive investigation and recording of evidence has to take both routes into consideration – from the point to the organ and from the organ to the point.

Changes in the Organ due to Stimulation of the Point

The first verification of the effect of acupuncture with Western medical methods (summarized by Bergsmann 1974) concerned point B 17, which is designated the point for the diaphragm, reunion of Yin and Yang, and master point of blood distribution. An effect on the working of the diaphragm is attributed to this point.

Under the precondition that there was a state of functional tension and no mechanical hindrance of the diaphragm, after stimulation of this point, which lies approximately in the region of the 7th thoracic vertebra, there was:

- relaxation of the diaphragmatic contour, and
- increase in diaphragmatic amplitude

In the first series, more than 200 patients were investigated by measuring diaphragmatic amplitude with serial radiographs of the diaphragm. The results were stereotyped. Occasional later observations gave the same results.

A single stimulus of point B 17 only gave a minimal effect on vital capacity and resistance. However, there was a reduction in expiratory reserve capacity corresponding to the relaxation of the thorax – the neutral respiratory position was displaced in the direction of expiration. Corresponding to the improved flexibility of the thorax, the inspiratory potentials of the intercostal muscles significantly increased in the electromyogram.

All findings, including muscle palpation, indicated relaxation of the thoracic movement system. This causes a reduction in respiratory work, and reduces the subjective sensation of dyspnea.

Starting from the observations on relaxation, we investigated the *dequi Sensation* of acupuncture. This was set of by a deep puncture in certain points that have a close relationship to muscle. The needle was stimulated mechanically or electrically, and a feeling of warmth combined with hypesthesia appeared in the direction of the target area.

We use points 3E 5–8, which have a close relationship to the finger and wrist extensors on the distal, dorsal lower arm, so that their stimulation activated the extension chain of the upper extremity.

Tab. 1: Results of investigation

	F	A	M. pectoralis F x A	F	A	M. trapezius F x A
Basic value Band relaxed	4.6	6.4	29.4	6.2	4.1	25.4
Fist	5.2	6.3	32.7	5.4	6.1	33.0
Dequi Hand relaxed	7.6	3.9	29.6	6.3	1.3	8.2
Fist	11.3	3.3	37.3	23.8	1.6	38.1

Wit the *EDP*-supported "Biofran" system (Schmidt Elektronik, Lindau, FRG), an electromyogram was taken of similarly long part of the pars horizontalis of the trapezius, which belongs to the extensor system, and pectoralis major, which partly belongs to the flexor chain.

Comparison parameters were the average frequency (F), the average amplitude (A), and the frequency-amplitude product, which were calculated and printed-out automatically. Preinvestigations had shown that the value with the greatest significance was F x A.

The results shown in Table 1 were taken from a series of 11 analogously-running myographs. The investigation results show that F x A in the trapezius muscle, namely in the activated kinetic pathway chain, reduces significantly, while that in pectoralis major remains almost unaltered. Furthermore, the investigation shows that the effect is obtained through (peripheral) reduction of the amplitude, and that the centrally-regulated frequency remains unchanged. In dequi, deliberate fist clenching movement is only set off by frequency increase.

In this way, Western clinical methods verify that stimulation of certain points can alter the function of internal organs and muscles, and that there is a regulatory relationship between the point and the organ.

Alteration of the physical functions of the point in disease of the associated organ

Physical measurement results on neutral skin sites and at acupuncture points show highly inter-individual and situation-related distribution. As a result of the large number of variants, which, not unusually, are not related to the clinical analysis, an inter-individual comparitive investigation

has little chance of success. This is also not needed in the diagnosis of individual regulatory behaviour. The questions are:
- What ist the initial state of the patient and/or his organs?
- How is a test stimulation of the ground system carried out?
- From this, conclusions can be made on the function of the ground system.

To understand the functioning process of the ground system through a local process, value differences have to be understood as an expression of *"regulatory disintegration"*, and this permits conclusions to be made about the status of the ground system and its reaction capacity.

The ground system is open in the area where regulation is not affected, and is thus reactive and capable of regeneration. However, under the influence of patho-information proceeding from the process, a "regulatory compartment" uncoupled from macroorganic regulation is formed, where stimuli receive either a labile-excessive or sluggish response, or no response.

In a state of general stress to the patient, only the stimulus response and the functional capacity of the ground system tested by this can give information about the ground system status.

Finally, this variation in stimulus response depends on the ground substances structures being loaded with electrical charges but for verification we have to await the results of future histochemical and histophysical investigations.

Phenomena in the Acupuncture Point that can be Palpated

Palpation finds changes in the consistency and elasticity of tissue, namely physical qualities. Since it is the method most frequently used in practice, the results should be taken as the start-point.

The palpatory symptoms in the active point are:
- Stereotype situation in relation to muscles, tendons, periosteum and fascia
- With surface palpation, the point presents as a flat depression where the skin relief is smoother.
- The skin over the point is less mobile – "the finger stays put".
- With greater pressure the muscle under the point is felt to be significantly harder.

- In the center, a tender cord with a small node can be felt
- The point is more sensitive to pain.
- With mechanical stimulation of the point, referred pain is set-off in a distant reference zone, but this always lies in the kinetic chain of the muscle.
- These symptoms are not present in non-stressed muscles.

It seems significant that even with simple assessment of the point qualities by palpation, the regulatory processes at the point can be diagnosed, for the non-stressed – inactive – point is not palpable, while the activated point – with regulatory change – can be found by palpation.

Since the point qualities can alter in seconds, palpatory control of therapy is also possible.

Thermal Phenomena

Our thermal tests were carried out with the Medical IR-Thermometer from the Barnes Company (Conn., USA). Analogous results can also be obtained with contact thermometry. We prefer the IR method because it works without contact and thus without additional stimulation.

Steady-state investigations for the comparison of "free" and "stressed" points. Acupuncture point Lu 8 was used, which lies at the level of the radial apophysis, over the radial artery. The subjects were patients with severe unilateral tuberculosis processes in the lung.

Table 2 shows clearly that the average values in both patient groups only differ in distribution. However, the difference between free point and stressed point for the two groups differs with 5% probability of error. In the active processes, the stressed point is 0.45 degrees warmer, and in the inactive processes 0.45 degrees cooler than its free counterpart.

Tab. 2: Comparison of IR radiation of point Lu 8 (in degrees C) n = 20

	free side	stressed side	difference
Inactive process	32.45	32.0	– 0.45
Active process	31.5	31.95	+ 0.45
Difference	0.95 (t)	0.05 ns	0.9 s

Thermoregulatory tests

The behaviour of the thermic side differences – thermoregulatory disintegration – was investigated with cooling of both hands, to obtain insight into the thermoregulatory capacity in various diseases. The difference between the point and neutral skin on the stressed side and the difference between the stressed point and free point was recorded graphically. The resulting curves indicate maximal labile behaviour in the active process and dampening of regulatory behaviour in the healthy one.

Electrophysiological Phenomena

Conductance investigations

After preliminary investigations with various measurement systems, which established that there is a positive potential and increased conductance on the side of the process in chronically ill patients, systematic investigations were carried out with an instrument designed by *Woolley-Hart* (*Bergmsann* and *Woolley-Hart*, 1973). This instrument permitted an increase in voltage in 0.5 V steps and made it possible to measure the resulting current in micro A. There was an almost linear increase in the lower voltage stages, corresponding to Ohm's Law, up to individually varying high voltage, from where the current began to rise with a steeper gradient or in a curve. This voltage was termed the breaking point, and showed itself to be the most useful comparison parameter for our investigations.

In connection with this investigation, *Maresch* constructed a voltage ramp that rose from 0 to 12 V in 50 s, and then regressed. The resulting current was recorded as a hysteresis curve. In this type of test, the breaking point could not be defined clearly, and could only be estimated. The most useful value was 12 volt current (or, possibly, 9 volts) and the maximal hysteresis (*Bergsmann* 1974).

In all investigations, the values at the activated point were compared with the free point and neutral skin sites.

The comparative values shown in Tab. 3 concern point Lu 8, which has a close relationship to the thorax and is found at the level of the radial apophysis above the radial artery.

Tab. 3: I/E measurement at Lu 8 – parameter micro A

	free side		stressed side		
	Lu 8	i. H.	Lu 8		i. H.
unilateral minor lung bk. n = 8	2.3 ↑ s ↓	1.9 ↑ s ↓	1.8	← t →	1.1
unilateral major lung bk. n = 10	0.8 ↑	0.7 _____ s _____	1.4 ↑	← s →	0.7

The comparisons shown in Tab. 4 concern point Lu 9, which has an intensive relationship with the liver and is found at the level of the medial knee joint fold.

Tab. 4: I/E measurement at Lu 9 – parameter micro A

	left side		right side	
	Lu 9	i. H.	Lu 9	i. H.
Healthy liver n = 12	2.2	1.6	2.1	1.5
Liver disease n = 15	6.7	3.8	13.3	6.2

Both investigations clearly show that the function of the ground system is altered measureably at the point through homolateral processes, and that through this conclusions can be made on the state of the body region from the function at the point, with which it can be brought into relationship according to the rules of acupuncture.

The automatically produced I/E curves are well suited to investigations on the trunk. Here too, significant differences between the point and neutral skin could be established unilaterally, and the point over the process and the contralateral point. At the same time we found a significant dorsal-ventral difference, corresponding to the tomographically-verified lung process.

Further investigations showed that an effective acupuncture is suitable for balancing the measured values between the points, and, at the same time, for normalizing the values. However, in these investigations we had to take into account the fact that in longer-lasting investigations, the bioelectric properties of the points are altered by orthostatic processes, which are unavoidable with prolonged sitting or standing. We followed this further in a personal trial program, and were able to establish this with all points, particularly those of the lower extremities. These events were particularly those of the lower extremities. These events were particularly obvious with varicose legs. On the other hand, we found that the electrical substantiation of the reaction to minimal stimulus levels is only possible while sitting, namely with reduced orthostasis.

Recent investigations carried out with a modern, completely automatic measuring instrument (Name of the prototype: *Impulse Dermotest*) confirm our previous findings.

Potential Difference Investigations

We evaluate the local potentials and the resulting potential differences as the primary bioelectrical variables. They are also, to this extent, to be regarded as a connection between biophysics and biochemistry, as every chemical process also alters the local charge relationships. Variations, perfusion, alter current potentials. Physical-chemical influences vary membrane potentials, and every stimulus is accompanied by metabolic changes that lead to local potential displacements. External electrical and magnetic fields produce dipolar molecules, whose polarization also influences the local potentials. In sum, these and other factors are part of the measurement of local potential, and, as a result, determine the local potential difference. The strengths of the fields resulting from the charges lead to charge displacements and ion wandering in the ground system, and determine its functional state. Seen in this way, potential differences are in the center point of the physico-chemical events.

In both palms and point Lu 8 on the side of chronic lung processes we always found positive potentials as compared to the contralateral side; in indurative processes, the process side was negatively charged in comparison to the contralateral side.

Recently, we have investigated this phenomenon with the *Impulse Dermotest* instrument already mentioned. Using this method, the potential differences between the electrodes are measured 4 times, and the conductance value is measured between every two potential measurements. In this way, a native potential and its alterations is recorded through the charge flow and the conductance measurement. Since every foreign current alters the bioelectrical status of the measurement site, this method can be evaluated as a standard bioelectrical regulation test.

The following results were obtained from 25 subjects with subclinical, but palpable tension in the upper and lower arm. The measurement point was the trigger of the extensor carpi radialis muscle, which corresponds to AP Di 10. Table 5 shows that a lower potential is measured in an subclinically tensed muscle than in its relaxed counterpart.

Tab. 5: M extensor carpi radialis

PD	tensed arm	free arm	diff
MW in mV	104 mV	119.34 mV	14.78
Strg.	79.00	64.12	8.7

It must be emphasized that these subjects with subclinical tension had no feeling of tension and no pain.

In the following, rehabilitation patients with unilateral tension pain were investigated, and the potentials at the painful APs in the tension area were compared with those at the symmetrically-inactive point. Naturally, the site of the counterelectrode was not altered. Table 6 gives the results from 19 double measurements.

Tab. 6: Point measurement – potentials

active points	N = 19	inactive points
P 1 – 95 +, – 67 mV		– 58 +, – 48 mV
P 2 – 134 +, – 48 mV		– 107 +, – 65 mV
P 3 – 130 +, – 53 mV		– 129 +, – 63 mV
P 4 – 134 +, – 62 mV		– 152 +, – 60 mV
paracomparison for P1		
D = 37		
sD = 17.64		
t = 2.1206, p > 0,05		

Apart from the significantly lower primary potential, it is noticeable that the potentials at the pain points (current measurement) have significantly less alteration than the control points.

Comparative electromyographical investigations with standardized isometric stress have shown that a significantly higher frequency-amplitude product in the tensed muscle than in muscle with normal tone. This leads to the question of whether the potentials in the overlying points are altered by the action potentials of the musculature directly, or via tension states in the fascia and the resulting perfusion change in the point area.

Conclusions on the local state of function of the matrix can also be made, and here we see an indication of depolarization processes and a reduction of biophysical (and biochemical) reaction capacity. Both are symptoms of regulatory disintegration.

Harmonization of Rhythm

Recently, we have found the previously unknown effect of point stimulation; through needling and laser radiation of a point in muscle groups in functional relationship to the rules of acupuncture, the previously disarranged frequency spectrum program is brought into harmony.

Equipment and Methods

The EDP-supported 2 canal amplification system from Schmidt Electronics (Lindau) is used. The computer program processes the raw potentials of the musculature taken from surface electrodes, and gives the average frequency, amplitude, and the frequency-amplitude product. In addition, a Fourier analysis of 1–33 Hz can be called-up.

Patients with a variety of tension and tension pain symptoms in the tension area were myographied, using a standardized isometric stress. The investigation was repeated during and after a variety of therapeutic methods.

Results

The changes in the Fourier frequency spectrogram brought about by acupuncture and laser therapy were interesting. While there was previously no noticeable regulation in the sequence of maximal and minimal frequencies, during and after the therapy wave-shaped sequences in 4–7 Hz stages could be seen.

This corresponds to the total harmonic relationship of higher range of acoustics.

Observation of this phenomenon was not limited to treatment of points situated near the symptom area. It was also observed in radiation or needling of far distant points (e.g. the ankle in shoulder symptoms). However, it could not be achieved through treating points that had no relationship to the target area according to the rules of acupuncture, and also not by treatment of neutral skin areas.

This investigation shows that stimulation of a point with two different qualities has a regulatory effect on the rhythmic relationships of the organism. Also, when the participation of rhythmogenetic centers does not come into the question, it has to be assumed that the ground system participates in the perception and transmission of frequencies, as a structure capable of oscillation. It is also probable that it is capable of altering mechanical stimuli to oscillations.

The appearance of total harmonious regulation under the influence of acupuncture, or treatment with electromagnetic fields (lasers), indicates a problem that has been generally ignored in medicine up to now – the harmonious regulation of host rhythms; according to *Hildebrandt* (1972) these have a total interrelationship. Our investigations show that this regulation can also be demonstrated in the frequency mixture in somatic muscle. It appears to be damaged by pathological hypertonicity and to reappear with effective therapy.

Synopsis

In the sense of continuing clinical-practical ground system research, the acupuncture point can be regarded as the

Window to the Ground System

Palpatory, thermic and electrical measurement series on a variety of points have shown that a good insight into the functional state and the regulatory potency of the ground system can be obtained in the test. In this connection, the recording of potential differences has special significance, since conclusions on the molecular charge can be made from them.

The relationships to rhythmogenesis require further investigation.

Diagnostic Methods

First of all an emphatic warning: all the methods described here give *reflex-regulatory* results, which can not give evidence about the possible presence of pathomorphology; they can only give evidence on *functional* states. They therefore have to be regarded as screening or a *complement* to normal clinical diagnosis with imaging methods and biochemical parameters.

Palpation of Clinical Signs Caused by Reflexes

This concerns more than the usual palpation of pathomorphologies in clinical medicine; it concerns the establishment of reflectory changes in the skin, subcutaneous tissue and muscle. Various strengths of palpation are used in layers to register the reflexly-addressed areas, but always with the least possible pressure. The dermatome system and knowledge of the kinetic chains simplify the allocation of the findings to specific organs. The systematics of the reflex pathological signs of internal organs and the organs of the movement apparatus is known (*Bergsmann* and *Bergsmann* 1988), but their description would exceed the parameters of this book.

Palpation is the most useful method in daily medical practice, and its results differ from those obtained from methods supported by instruments by less than 5%. An experienced practitioner can also use palpation in the field of focal diagnosis, since minimal lasting stress to a focus (e.g. tooth or tonsil), like other processes, leads to palpable changes in the appropriate reflex zones.

Thermodiagnosis, Infrared Diagnosis

Thermodiagnosis is one of the oldest medical examination methods. The infrared radiation diagnostic methods developed in recent decades, and the development of the thermistor sensor, as well as the improvement of the bimetal feeler brought the possibility of rapid and exact diagnostic procedures to this field, as well as the possibility of computer-supported evaluation of the results.

Contact thermometry only registers the temperature differences; which are actuated due to the regulatory disintegration of reflexly affected skin areas and non-stimulated skin areas on the one hand, and between neutral skin and the point on the other. Here, the measurement in steady state has significantly less to say than the test of function; namely, the measurements before and after a cooling stimulus, and the type of reaction is evaluated according to the stimulus.

Since infrared radiation outside the 4th potency of absolute temperature is also determined by a skin radiation coefficient, IR diagnosis has to be regarded more differentially, and it also makes more extensive diagnostic statements than contact thermometry possible. Changes in the radiation coefficient are mainly caused by the CO_2 content of the vascular bed and by changes in skin relief. It is true that the latter cannot be evaluated as a variation in radiation properties, but smoothing of the skin surface causes less radiation per surface unit, while microfoldings cause an increase per surface unit. However, since the structure of the skin surface is generally under autonomic control, this variation concerns a regulatory system that involves much more than the question of temperature.

Information on the measuring systems and further literature can be found in *Blohmke* (1979) and *Heim* for IR diagnosis, and in *Rost* for thermodiagnosis.

Electrodiagnosis

Only a few bioelectrical parameters and their changes are registered and evaluated with currently available electrodiagnostic methods:

- the conductance (reciprocal resistance)

- the potential difference between the electrodes and

- the capacity of the tissue

Recently, the establishment of host oscillations and their changes was added to the above. This is not the place to make an evaluation or to describe details of methodology, but the main principles and their physiological basis should be mentioned.

The Electro Skin Test

This method is concerned with over-threshold stimulation of the skin with galvanic power. In reflex-affected projection zones and maximal points there is livid reddening, which lasts longer then in non-affected skin. This method, which is also termed electropalpation is mainly found to be unpleasant and painful on sensitive skin.

Conductance Measurement

The first systematic measurements of conductance were undoubtedly carried out by *Regelsberger* sen. in the dermatomes of diseased organs. However, since then, point measurement for diagnostic purposes has experienced a great expansion, and the deviation of the conductance upwards from a system-dependent *standard value* is evaluated as a sign of hyperergia (irritation, inflammation, allergy), while the deviation downwards is interpreted as hypoergia (degeneration, regulatory blockade, exhaustion). The measurements are taken at a variety of acupuncture points – mainly at the endpoints of the meridians in the fingers and toes. In addition, there are other points in the fingers and toes that are not used in acupuncture. The localization of a disturbance or disease is diagnosed according to the rules of acupuncture and the allocation of points to organs. *Here from personal observations, the movement apparatus and its multiple possibilities for disturbances are underrated.*

Measurement of Potential Difference

The diagnostic evaluation of potential differences is mainly neglected in practical electrodiagnosis, although the changes in potential are mainly the primary electrical deviation in disturbances of function and disease, which often lead to secondary changes in the conductance. Up to now, this measurement has been integrated into only two diagnostic methods; one of these is suitable for point measurements (Impulse Dermotest) and the other for bioelectrical diagnostic review (BF Decoder).

Measurement of Capacity

The capacity of tissue can be measured; a defined tension is expressed over a previously determined period of time, then the reverse flow from the tissue is recorded with short circuit switching. The various participating biological components have to be taken into account in the evaluation, for this investigation is accompanied by a variety of bioelectrical phenomena, such as taking-up electrons, ion wandering and polarization processes in fixed dipolar molecules.

Measurement of Host Electromagnetic Signals

Apart from such clinically established methods such as EEG, ECG, EMG, etc., there have been more and more attempts to register host electromagnetic signals in recent years, and to evaluate them from the diagnostic point of view. Up to now, none of these systems has reached the point where it can be recommended for practical application, especially as the interpretation of the results varies from investigator to investigator, and, due to this, it is not unusual that they are subject to criticism. However, one should bear in mind the resonance capacity of organic structures, and that new physiological and pathological knowledge can be certainly be expected from their investigation (*Bergsmann* 1983).

Regulatory Therapy

The primary aim of regulatory therapy is to restore disturbed regulatory mechanisms to normal, namely to restore the optimal regulatory state, and to guarantee the homeostasis and economcy of the organism in this way. Treatments that have a positive effect on regulation can be combined optimally with clinical forms of therapy, provided that the latter do not produce an additional regulatory stress, such as high doses of corticoids and psychopharmaceutics.

The most, important points in regulatory therapy are:

1. Overcoming factors that disturb regulation, such as minimal chronic stress, heavy metal load, consumption of luxury poisons, excess nutrition, etc.

2. The balancing-out of possible deficiencies that lead to regulatory dysfunction, such as deficiencies of vitamins, ferments, trace elements, etc.

3. Breaking down pathogenic feedback mechanisms, for example with acupuncture and/or neural therapy, and also with stimulation therapy.

4. It also seems to be possible today to carry out specific regulatory therapy with resonance to electromagnetic impulses, but the indications and possibilities have not yet been fully investigated.

It is not possible to give a description of all the possibilities in this book, but it is simple to give a place to each of the special techniques that have been enummerated.

Literature

Athenstaedt, H.: Pyroelectric and piezoelektric properties of vertebrates. An. New York Acad. sc. Vol. **238,** 68 (1974).

Bergsmann, O.: Begünstigen banale extrapulmonale Herde homolateralen Beginn der Lungentuberkulose? Beitr. Klin. Tbk. 125, 506 (1963).

–: Akupunktur als Problem der Regulationsphysiologie. Karl F. Haug Verlag. Heidelberg 1974.

–: *Damböck, E., Glaser, M., Puchas, A.:* Der banale extrapulmonale Herd als Gestaltungsfaktor der Lungentuberkulose. Praxis der Pneumologie 22. 3. 1968.

–: Bioelektrische Funktionsdiagnostik. Karl F. Haug Verlag. Heidelberg 1979.

–: Über muskuläre Resonanz- und Dämpfungsphänomene bei Akupunktur und Lasertherapie. DZA 3 (1985).

–: Vertebro-respiratorische und vertebro-zirkulatorische Syndrome als leistungsbegrenzende Faktoren bei Degenerationsleiden des Bewegungsapparates. Rheuma 2 (1986).

–: Störfeldpathogenese und Realität des Sekundenphänomens. Rheuma 2 (1987).

–: *Woolley-Hart, A.:* Differences in Electrical Skin Conductivity between Acupuncturepoints and adjacent Skin Areas. Am. J. Acupuncture 1, 27 (1973).

–: *Bergsmann, R.:* Projektionssymptome – reflektorische Krankheitszeichen. Universitätsverlag Facultas. Wien 1988.

–: Elektromyografische Verifizierung der postisometrischen Relaxation bei peripheren Spannungssymptomen. Manuelle Medizin 1988.

–: *Eder, M.:* Funktionelle Pathologie und Klinik der Brustwirbelsäule. G. Fischer Verlag. Stuttgart 1982.

–: *Meng, A.:* Akupunktur und Bewegungsapparat – Versuch einer Synthese. Karl F. Haug Verlag. Heidelberg 1982.

Blohmke, M.: Klinische Überprüfung der Thermoregulationsdiagnostik. Phys. Med. und Rehab. 7 (1979).

Brückle, G.: Intravitalmikroskopische Untersuchungen über Aufbau und Hämodynamik der normalen terminalen Strombahn der Unterlippenschleimhaut des Menschen. Inauguraldissertation 1963.

Brügger, A.: Die Erkrankungen des Bewegungsapparates und seines Nervensystems. G. Fischer Verlag. Stuttgart 1980.

Drischel, H.: Einführung in die Biokybernetik. Akademie Verlag. Berlin 1973.

Gleditsch, J. M.: Reflexzonen und Somatotopien. WBV Schorndorf 1983.

Fröhlich, K.: zitiert nach *Popp.* Vortrag an der Jahrestagung der DAH, Bad Nauheim 1984.

Hansen, K., Schliack, H.: Segmentale Innervation, ihre Bedeutung für Klinik und Praxis. G. Thieme Verlag. Stuttgart 1963.

Head, H.: Sensibilitätsstörungen der Haut bei Viszeralerkrankungen. Hirschwald Verlag. Berlin 1898.

Heine, H.: siehe Beitrag *Heine.*

Hildebrandt, G.: Therapeutische Physiologie, Grundlagen der Kurortbehandlung in Balneologie. Medizinische Klimatologie. Springer Verlag. Heidelberg 1985.

Keidel, W.: Lehrbuch der Physiologie. G. Thieme Verlag. Stuttgart 1970.

Klima, H.: Dissertation (Exp. Physik). Wien 1981.

–: Unbeachtete Informationssysteme des Organismus; vorgetragen am Symp. d. österr. Ges. f. Neuralth. Baden bei Wien 1987.

Mackenzie, J.: Krankheitszeichen und ihre Auslegung. Kabitzsch Verlag. Würzburg 1911.
Nordenström, B. E. W.: Biologically closed electric circuits. Nordic Medical Publications 1983.
Perger, F.: siehe Beitrag *Perger.*
Popp, F. A.: Biophotonen. 2., verb. u. erw. Aufl. Verlag für Medizin Dr. Ewald Fischer GmbH, Heidelberg 1984.
–: Neue Horizonte in der Medizin. 2., erw. Aufl. Karl F. Haug Verlag. Heidelberg 1988.
Ricker, G.: Pathologie als Naturwissenschaft. Springer Verlag. Berlin 1924.
Travell, J. G., Simons, D. G.: Myofascial pain and dysfunction. Williams & Wilkins. Baltimore/London 1983.
Zwiener, U.: Pathophysiologie neurovegetativer Regelungen und Rhythmen. G. Fischer Verlag. Jena 1976.

(Prim. Univ.-Doz. Dr. med. Otto Bergsmann, Auhofstraße 37, A-1130 Wien)

Part Three

Therapeutic Consequences of Ground Regulation Research

The Puncture Phenomenon

For *Pischinger* it was always a special concern to point out that even minor injuries like a puncture with a needle – whether for taking blood, acupuncture or neural therapy, lead to significant reactions in the extracellular matrix. This is discussed below.

Normally, taking blood leads to major changes in iodine consumption, *Pischinger* (1975) emphasized that the loss of 3–5 ml blood cannot be made responsible for this phenomenon. Only the puncture itself comes into the question; it affects the perivascular tissue; soft connective tissue with a rich supply of autonomic nerves. I have therefore referred to the puncture phenomenon or the puncture effect. The puncture produces a wound, although a small one (*Kellner* 1971, Kellner u. *Feucht* 1969), which – as will be discussed in detail later – lies in the range that can be measured.

This puncture effect is also manifested in other autonomic functions, and is an essential, item in the non-specific range. This will be described in more detail below, and confirmed by trial results.

At first, a few examples of the phenomenon of results in iodometry. We have, of course, to understand the processes involved in puncturing the vein precisely. The puncture penetrates the skin epithelium, the connective tissue of the papillary layer, the firm tissue of the stratum textosum with extracellular tissue spread along nerves and vessels, the perivascular tissue, which also has extracellular tissue, the muscular wall of the vein, and then the intima and the blood. This means that there are more than enough places where the autonomic reflexes can be stimulated; starting in particular from the perivascular system, which contains the triad for ground regulation – including extracellular fluid (see the skin investigations carried out by G. *Kellner* 1966).

The puncture with an injection or acupuncture needle works in three ways: firstly through the smallest injury causing the longest-lasting effect (according to *Kellner* and *Feucht* (1969) at least five days), secondly due to the temperature difference between the needle and the tissue (needle at room temperature of between 20° and 22°, tissue at between 36° and 37°), and thirdly due to the potential difference between tissue and needle, which can be measured, according to *Bethe* (1952), *Gildemeister* (1928), *Hauswirth* (1953), *Kracmar* (1961), *Neuberger* (1960), *Croon* (1976) and *Maresch* (1970). Electrical stimuli spread very rapidly through the ground system of the entire organism. A photon emission from injured or dying cells reaches the neighbouring cells in 10^{-7} seconds, and spreads throughout the entire organism with the speed of sound (*Popp* 1984).

Kellner (1971) and *Bergsmann* (1965) have confirmed the effects of the temperature difference, using an infrared camera and with rheography respectively.

Figs. 1 and 2 show a series of puncture reactions in diagrammatic form (*Pischinger* 1975). The individual initial values are at different levels. Related to a "zero point", they show extraordinary differences in reaction pattern. The reason for this is the individual defence state of the subjects. These results can be used to test the defence state.

The reaction of a healthy subject corresponds to *Selye's* (1953) *alarm reaction, a stimulus of this size is completely adjusted-out within 3 to 4 hours. In the first hour the iodine consumption value in Pischinger's iodometry sinks, returning to the initial value in the following 2 to 3 hours.* One can speak of a shock and countershock reaction.

Disturbed reactivity of the nonspecific system leads to other reaction forms (RF), but these are subject to certain natural laws; major excesses in iodine consumption values (ICV) appear in diseases of the immediate allergy type, and under certain conditions the puncture reaction can trigger an asthma attack. A reduction in the ICV is seen in diseases of the delayed allergy type (e.g. inflammatory rheumatic disease, multiple sclerosis, ulcerative colitis, etc. In consumptive diseases there is no reaction (e.g. malignancies, leukemia, thorotrast damage, and also the late and final stages of inflammatory diseases like tuberculosis or chronic-progressive systemic diseases).

It is clear from this test group that the nonspecific system reacts extremely sensitively. The puncture itself triggers the reaction; in this case with the iodine consumption values. The skeptical question has been posed several times; why doesn't the puncture for the second blood sample triggers a reaction analogous to the first one? One dare not ignore the fact that an

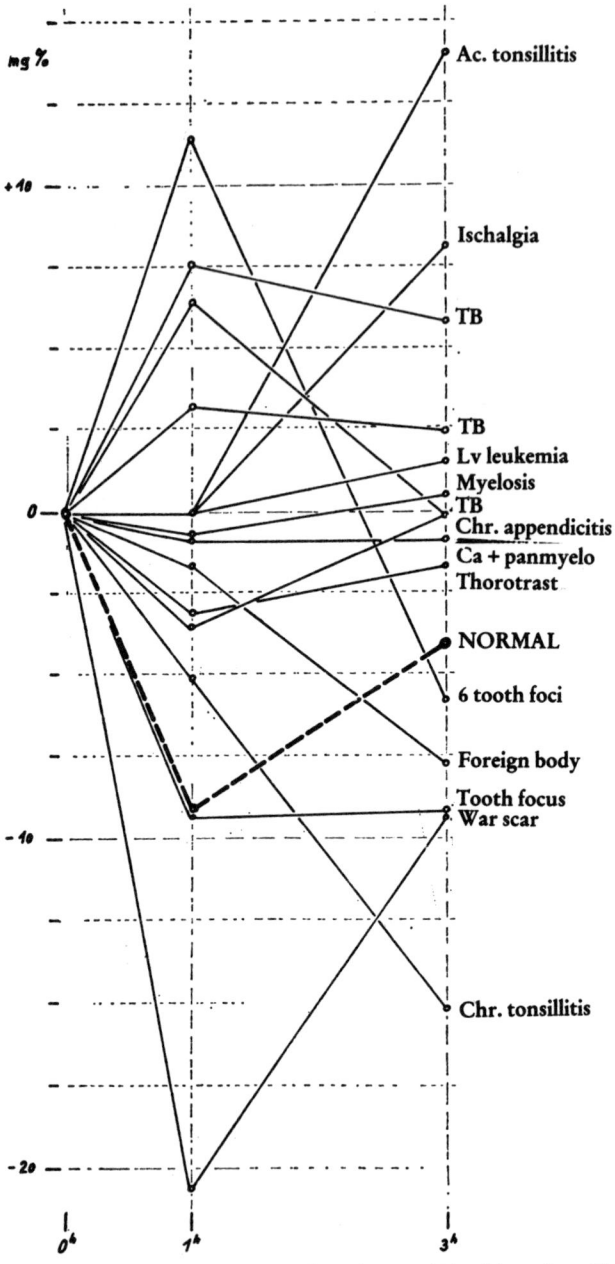

Fig. 1: Types of reaction in a 3 hour stress test after taking 5 ml blood from the cubital vein. All initial values are entered as 0, and the deviations in the succeeding hours as + or – values in mg% iodine utilization. Abscissa: time after taking blood in hours.

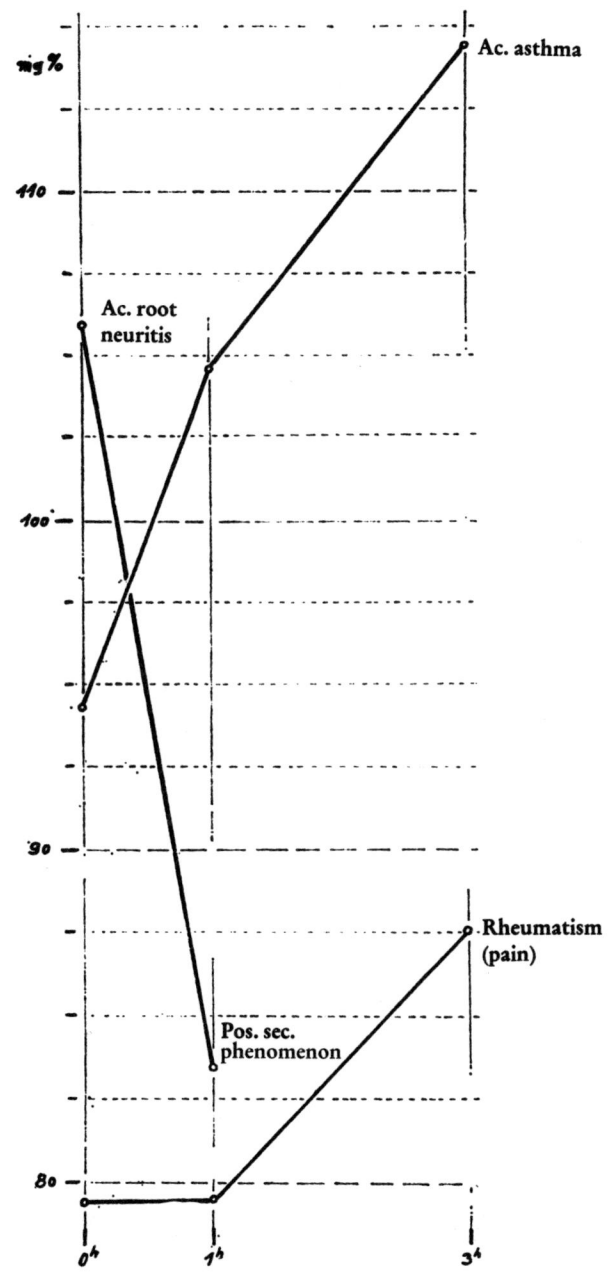

Fig. 2: Puncture effect. Acute attacks of asthma or ischias are initiated with the increase in IUV. Scar infiltration with Impletol produces a reduction in the raised IUV and easing of pain in acute root neuritis (secondary phenomenon)

organism does not react to further autonomic influences during an alarm reaction – as extensive investigations by *Lickint* (1923) and *Selye* (1952) have shown.

However, the investigations also show that the reaction state of an organism can be tested from the physico-chemical characteristics of a protein-free or protein-poor serum extract if it has been obtained with care, and the defence and reaction capacities from standardized mild stresses, such as the puncture. It is obvious that this concerns a humoral reaction which, however, cannot develop without the other nonspecific areas of the autonomic system. It should be mentioned here in passing that this is the basic phenomenon of *acupuncture*.

However, the most important point seems to be the fact that even the most minor irritation of the tissue in question, or a puncture, triggers the entire reaction system – here, the nonspecific ground regulation system is meant in particular, *Pischinger refers to a puncture phenomenon that manifests the totality character of the ground system.*

Tab. 1

	Time	Erythro.	Leuko	Segm.	Eo.	Baso.	Mono.	Lympho.	Disint
I	8	5 320 000	8 366	5 020	250	0	500	2 430	160
	9	5 370 000	8 832	4 240	179	88	353	3 000	972
	11	4 800 000	6 978	3 980	69	69	628	2 023	209
II	8	4 400 000	4 100	2 255	41	41	164	1 435	164
	9	4 330 000	4 000	2 160	40	40	160	1 400	200
	11	4 200 000	4 100	2 091	41	41	164	1 435	328
III	8	–	5 100	2 300	50	50	150	2 000	550
	9	–	4 466	1 700	45	90	135	1 956	540
	11	–	6 400	2 956	0	64	320	2 100	960

Tab. 2

Skin	R	C		
undamaged	1.30	0.069		
1 puncture point	1.75	0.07973	R	in kiloohms
3 puncture points	2.11	0.145	C	in microfarad
7 puncture points	1.76	0.380		
14 puncture points	1.33	0.940		

Tab. 3

Patient	Day of measurement	Time of measurement	Initial state		Puncture reaction	
			R	C	R	G
Dita Sch.	1. 3. 69	8.35 Uhr	11.1	0.15	–	–
		12.20 Uhr	–	–	16.7	0.21
		12.23 Uhr	–	–	16.3	0.23
	5. 7. 69	8.35 Uhr	11.5	0.16	–	–
		12.20 Uhr	–	–	17.9	0.14
		12.23 Uhr	–	–	17.2	0.14
	8. 11. 69	8.35 Uhr	6.1	0.23	–	–
		12.53 Uhr	–	–	9.7	0.20
		12.55 Uhr	–	–	8.8	0.23
	16. 5. 70	8.10 Uhr	8.5	0.21	–	–
		12.25 Uhr	–	–	14.0	0.18
		12.27 Uhr	–	–	12.3	0.18
Josef Tr.	5. 7. 69	8.14 Uhr	6.3	0.23	–	–
		12.57 Uhr	–	–	9.5	0.25
		12.59 Uhr	–	–	6.7	0.29
	8. 11. 69	8.49 Uhr	5.4	0.27	–	–
		12.57 Uhr	–	–	3.2	0.31
		12.59 Uhr	–	–	2.9	0.44
Erna D.	5. 7. 69	8.35 Uhr	16.2	0.15	–	–
		12.47 Uhr	–	–	23.1	0.16
		12.49 Uhr	–	–	15.3	0.19
	8. 11. 69	8.43 Uhr	13.3	0.18	–	–
		12.52 Uhr	–	–	13.7	0.21
		12.54 Uhr	–	–	10.1	0.23
Peter J.	16. 5. 70	8.30 Uhr	13.3	0.12	–	–
		12.20 Uhr	–	–	24.1	0.10
		12.22 Uhr	–	–	16.1	0.14
Sr. Gebharda L.	16. 5. 70	8.50 Uhr	9.0	0.21	–	–
		12.29 Uhr	–	–	13.0	0.18
		12.31 Uhr	–	–	14.8	0.13

R in kiloohms
C in microfarad

These deviations from the normal reaction also show major differences in the extent of leukocyte breakdown (leukolysis). The simple puncture stimulus produces a more than quintuple increase in lysis forms than in healthy subjects (Tab. 1 *Pischinger* 1983). The humoral-autonomic blockade shown in case II (Tab. 2), only indicates an increase of 22% in lysis forms in the first hour, and of 100% after 3 hours – a greatly delayed and poor reaction, Case III reacts even more sluggishly and poorly: the lysis forms show no increase in the first hour; after three hours there is a minor increase of barely 70% (Tab. 3).

The significance of these variations was unclear. However, later investigations with simultaneous determination of immunoglobulins A, M and G gave three facts that make the significance of leukolysis for the defence system comprehensible:

1. The immunoglobulin changes (especially IgG) depend on the degree of leukolysis-minor leukolysis means a minor increase in the leukolysis rate, but a major increase in the immunoglobulins (particularly IgG), which indicates plasma cell breakdown;
2. Monocyte breakdown including release of triple-conjugated unsaturated fatty acids (*Pischinger's* factor M), which carry part of the responsibility for triggering humoral shock states and the switchover to the countershock reaction (the phase of immune system activity);
3. Granulocyte breakdown, which – as in the microphage phase of local defence – releases oxidative and proteolytic enzymes as well as interleukins, prostaglandins, and leukotrienes, and thus has an important role in the destruction of live microorganisms (*König* et al. 1988).

In the shock phase of the puncture reaction the ICV falls by about 10%, but by at least 50 μm/ml, returning to the initial value n the succeeding 3–4 hours.

However, reactions to the simple puncture are not only shown in iodometry and leukolysis; they are also shown in other nonspecific parameters, such as oxymetry of venous blood, in variations in minerals in situ and in venous blood, and even in the immunoglobulins of these take place sluggishly and are of longer duration.

The puncture also triggers bioelectrical changes.

Fig. 3: Puncture effect. Acute attacks of asthma or ischias are initiated with the increase in IUV. Scar infiltration with Impletol produces a reduction in the raised IUV and easing of pain in acute root neuritis (secondary phenomenon)

Polarization resistance   Polarization capacity

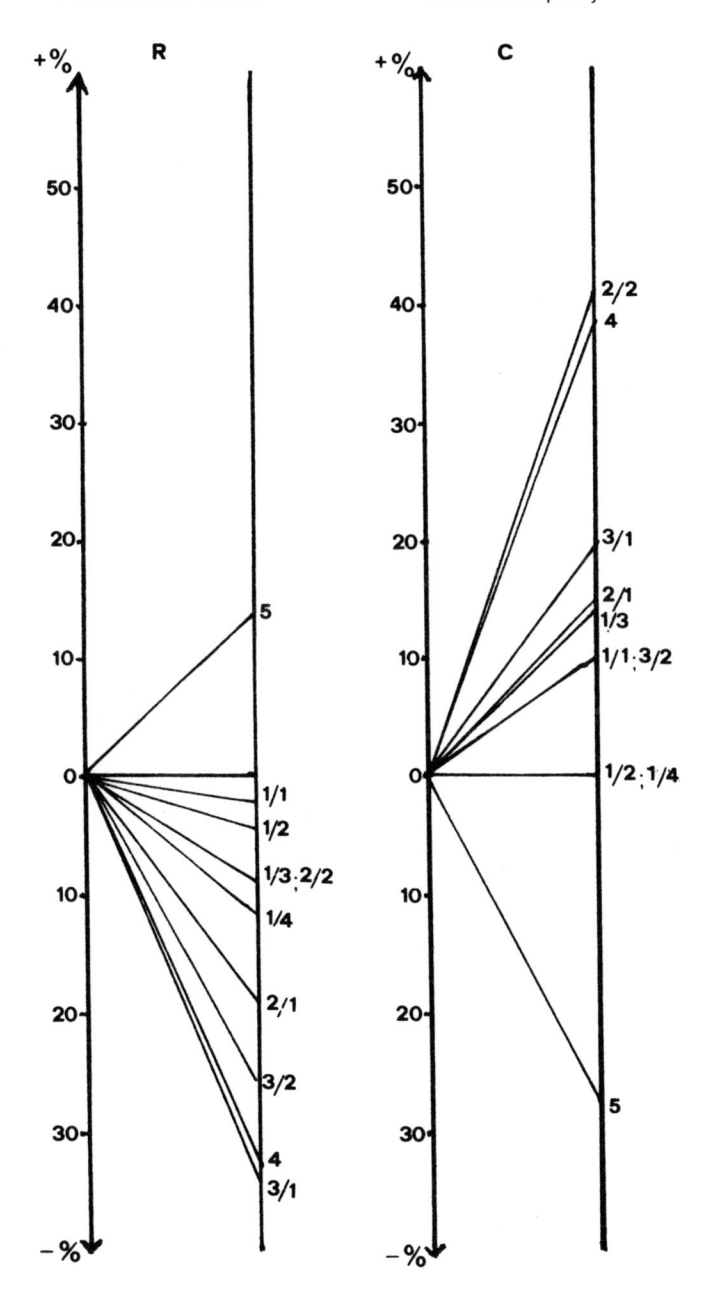

Bioelectrical Events with the Puncture Phenomenon

The bioelectrical phenomena in the puncture phenomenon indicate processes that are significant for the orientation of the defence state (*Pischinger* 1983).

As *Kracmar* (1971) reported, *Diehl* (1937) had already described changes in skin polarization values when needle punctures are made.

Gildemeister (1928) had already demonstrated that the polarization characteristics of the skin could be measured with a measuring bridge fed with alternating current.

Diehl (1937) used a 756 Hertz frequency; later, *Kracmar* (1971) used 50 Hertz, since with this method the polarization characteristics are seen more clearly, according to *Gerstner*, hand to hand resistance (R) is measured in kiloohms and capacity (C) in microfaradays (*Kracmar* 1971).

Here too, the type of reaction depends on the individual defence state existing at the time of the investigation, *Kracmar* established the same reactions with acupuncture needling.

These bioelectrical phenomena are accompanied by thermoregulatory changes. The skin temperature alters after needle punctures. *Kellner* (1971) was able to confirm this in acupuncture with an infrared camera. *Bergsmann* (1965) was also able to demonstrate the change in skin blood perfusion, using rheography.

These bioelectrical and thermoregulatory phenomena that take place when there is a puncture through the skin are important for characterization of the functions of the ground system. They indicate that biological reactions take place on the basis of electronic-energetic processes, and that there can be no life without these preconditions. Attention to morphological changes and purely biochemical processes has certainly brought much valuable knowledge, but it fails in the explanation of life itself, and, clinically more importantly, in the questions of energy and its activation in all living processes, including the defence functions.

If one bears in mind that each exogenous stimulus not only triggers cellular and humoral reactions, but is always accompanied by alterations in the biopotential, this is sufficient impetus to pay a great deal more attention now to these biopotentials than in the past. In addition, one must not become fixed on the point that these biophysical processes are absolutely necessary energetically for the diverse functional processes – but during cybernetic investigations it is more and more difficult to suppress this opinion and to refute it experimentally.

Warning must, however, be given about a great temptation. Again and again, one sees how direct specific diagnoses are drawn from such investigations, e.g. regarding silent inflammation, etc. This is false; it is true that decoder dermography and thermoregulatory diagnosis indicate the localization of a disturbance, but they cannot replace later specific diagnostic methods to determine the type of disturbance involved. They only document the state of the nonspecific system.

The entire significance and problems involved in the different bioelectrical processes is presented in a special contribution to this book by *Bergsmann*. It adopts the point of view that the puncture phenomenon is not only decisive in acupuncture, but also has an influence on neural therapy and every type of injection therapy – this opinion is also supported by the results from humoral investigations (e.g. the difference between injecting factor M and rubbing it in percutaneously). In addition, it should also be pointed out that even as a predominantly humoral medical practitioner one is confronted by the borderline reaction between biophysics and biochemistry in investigations concerning ground regulation, and expansion through biophysical knowledge is required to learn to understand the processes in chronic diseases. It can also be seen clearly in humoral research that every reaction that takes place in the borderline area between biophysics and biochemistry – e.g. oxygen consumption, the reactions in factor M according to *Pischinger*, in the electrolytes, etc. – take their course more rapidly and more sensitively than enzyme-controlled biochemical processes. These are facts that cannot be ignored.

Puncture Phenomenon and Oxygen Saturation of the Blood

Pischinger (1983) designates the alterability of the oxygen saturation of venous blood as the most important sign of the manifestation of the "totality reaction" in the ground functions.

It stands out that when venous blood is drawn the colour often varies between almost dark red and arterial bright red. The high degree of arterial coloration is particularly frequent during exacerbations of rheumatic inflammation and multiple sclerosis. This is certainly not always the case, but it is so frequent that this observation can be counted as a disturbance of oxygen consumption, which undoubtedly has significance in the disease picture (see also Chap. "Humoral Side Differences"). *Pischinger* (1954) began to follow up this phenomenon with an AO oxymeter (Hellige). Much later (1980–1986) it was possible to continue this in our own parameters, and his results were confirmed.

Basically, the puncture alone leads to the same reactions in oxygen consumption, i.e. the oxyhemoglobin content of venous blood, as in iodometry, leukolytic reaction and the R and C measurements, etc. Once again it was shown that the stimulus response depends on the individual defence situation at the time of the stimulus being given.

The many checks on the oxyhemoglobin content of venous blood in healthy subjects showed that at rest (at least 20 minutes before taking blood), it is about 40% (35–45%). The exogenous stimulus leads initially to an increase in venous blood oxyhemoglobin as a sign of a humoral-autonomic shock reaction. After 3 hours the stimulus is balanced-out and there is a return to the initial value. There are completely different initial

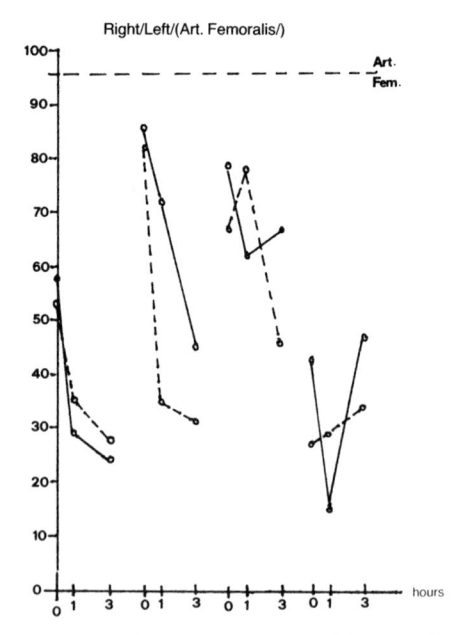

Fig. 4: Bilateral determination of O_2 contents. Solid line right, dotted line left vena cubitalis, 3- hour individual tests, asymmetrical reactions.

values in chronically ill patients. First of all, the frequently significantly increased oxyhemoglobin values in the exudative stages of inflammatory systemic diseases stand out, lying on average at 75%, but sometimes also reaching as much as 92%. If one considers that the oxyhemoglobin in the arterial limb of the vascular system is between 96% and 98%, such values show a significant reduction in oxygen delivery to the peripheral tissues. The reason for this could be an extreme opening of the arteriovenous anastomoses, which *Bergsmann* (1965) was able to demonstrate in his investigations on the blood perfusion of diseased organs. The puncture reaction temporarily reduces the blood perfusion even more. The reverse is found in chronically progressive inflammations, where there is increased oxygen consumption in the periphery; the oxyhemoglobin levels then reduce below the normal level of 40%; in extreme cases they can fall to 3% (!). This can also be explained by the work done by *Bergsmann*, which has already been mentioned. The sense of this extreme reversal of oxygen consumption in the periphery can only be answered hypothetically; in exudative disease processes, a higher oxygen content would probably be associated with massive tissue destruction, and would therefore be suppressed; in the chronic-progressive stage, however, there is a deficiency of energy, and there is an attempt to compensate for this by increased delivery and consumption. This assumption is based on the fact that the human organism is an open energy system (*Heine* 1987), subordinated to a biological flow balance with highly intermeshed regulatory systems (*v. Bertalanffy* 1975). Every organism is constantly striving to achieve this flow balance and also to obtain the necessary energy – there is therefore some justification for regarding the increased oxygen consumption as a substitute regulatory cycle for obtaining energy.

Iodometry and the Puncture Phenomenon

The results of iodometry according to *Pischinger*, which have already been described extensively in this book show that puncturing a vein produces the same response as a shock reaction. In healthy subjects there is a reduction of the ICV of at least 50 µg/ml. A counterregulation follows this fall in the first hour, leading to a restoration of the initial value in 3–4 hours. Patients with regulatory disturbances react significantly differently, and in a great variety of ways. Not only is the normal initial value of 810 µgICV greatly exceeded or reduced, variations (increase and reduction) differ greatly according to the type of progress the disease adopts, and the duration of the puncture reaction varies equally greatly.

Totality of Regulation in the Puncture Phenomenon

As *Pischinger* (1983) has already described, the puncture stimulus affects a series of characteristics of the humoral-autonomic field:
1. The differential blood count,
2. The number of leukocytes,
3. Iodometry,
4. Oxygen utilization in the periphery,
5. The skin electric parameters – clear reactions in the sense of the shock phase of an alarm reaction can be established in all these parameters; however, they depend on the individual initial state at the time,
6. *Pischinger* also puts forward the behaviour of the ground system in capillary microscopy (*Brückle* 1969).

The various types of reactions under differing initial situations also indicate that the highly intermeshed open energy system "human being" is primarily concerned with retaining life, and to prevent the possibly fatal effects of a direct, linear, cause-effect sequence. It is therefore impossible to establish such linear causalities, particularly in chronic diseases. One has to start from this premise to have any chance of understanding the various types of responses to stimuli, or to be able to give them due consideration.

Every stimulus that overcomes local defence triggers a reaction in the whole regulatory system and the entire intercellular-extracellular relations. It is very closely connected to all the other regulatory systems due to its close relationships (intermeshings) via the capillaries, the lymphatics and the autonomic nerve fibers. This leads to a *new* concept of the relative totality of functions in the organism, where the "sum" is greater than its parts.

The stimulation threshold for these totality reactions is, as shown by the puncture phenomenon, relatively low – it will be shown below that these thresholds can vary a great deal in sickness and in health. It is true that the reactions are total, but – and this was at first a surprise – they are not the same throughout the organism.

Testing the Initial State and Autonomic Asymmetry

Establishment of the defence reactions in chronic disease, particularly in inflammatory systemic diseases of unknown origin, was not only theroretically interesting, it brought advantages for therapy.

Initially efforts (*Perger* since 1949) were directed at establishing them through longitudinal hemograms on the progress of active disease processes, and, over a longer period, in the chronic-progressive forms of multiple sclerosis, and certain principles were actually found. However, the investigation conditions were very limited at that time (e.g. serum electrophoresis was only introduced in 1952). Initially, only the following measurements were possible; blood picture, and from this the absolute values for eosinophilic granulocytes, determination of the electrolyte value (Ca, Mg, later K), and the total cholesterol. It was known that Ca and the eosinophils play a role in allergies and allergy-type processes, and a paper by *Aiginger* (1951) on the variations in the Mg level in the active and interval stages of multiple sclerosis was available. However, even with these scanty means it was possible to establish the most important types of reaction in the exacerbations and chronic-progressive course of multiple sclerosis and the significantly different reactions of these parameters in acute febrile reactions; the latter in an influenza epidemic in 1954.

Initially, three of the possible types of reaction were established: the normal, strong reaction of a healthy defence system in acute infections

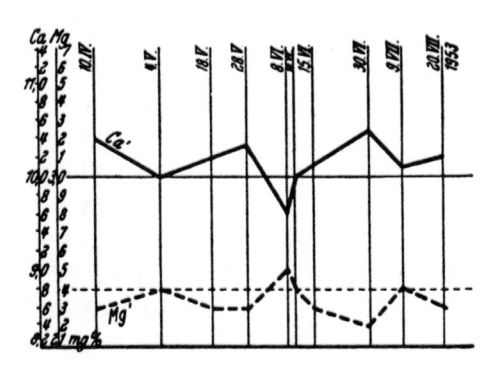

Fig. 5A: Ca-Mg curves in a case of inpatient MS (normergic reaction). Ca —, Mg ——— (the thin lines with Ca, 10.0 mg%, with Mg 2.4 mg% give the critical level of the ion values (see text).

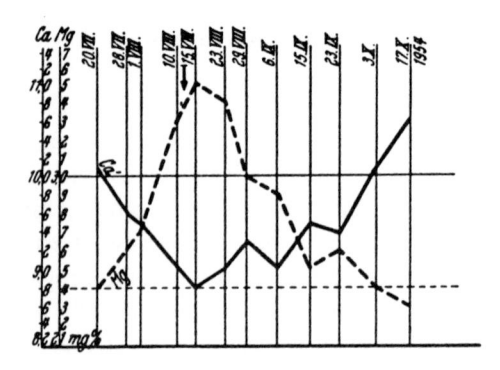

Fig. 5B: Typical Ca-Mg curves before and during an exacerbation. From 26.7.54 subj. complaints, malaise, insomnia. First clinical symptoms on 13.8.54; on 23.8.54 symptoms static, with subsequent remission.

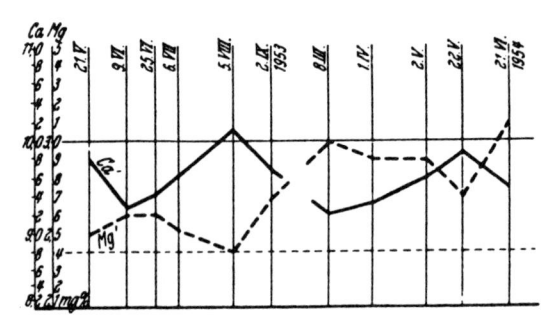

Fig. 5C: Longitudinal section of Ca-Mg levels in chronic-progressive MS, observed for 1 year. Ca remains under 10.0 mg% and Mg above 2.4%.
(Fig. 5 from: *Perger*, DMW 81 [1956] 342 [Allergy Supplement])

also showed the possibility of interpreting the findings. It showed rapid and extensive variations in the electrolytes, with some minor subsequent variations in the electrolytes, with some minor subsequent variations in convalescence. This corresponded to *the alarm reaction that had just been described by Selye* (1952), with shock, countershock and reconvalescence phases. The total duration lay between 7 and 10 days, and the total range of deviation lay at about 40% in the changeover from the shock to the antishock phase.

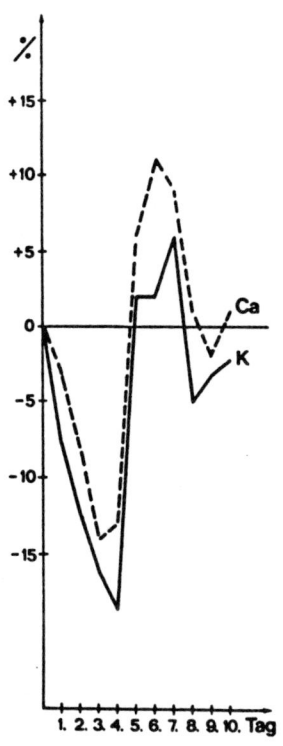

Fig. 6: Variations in electrolyte values (mg%) in percent of the initial value in acute infection. (from: *Perger*, Vienna, Med. WS 128 [1978] 31–37)

Nothing of this reactive triad was noticed in the exacerbations of multiple sclerosis. The entire clinical progress was accompanied by an electrolyte picture that corresponded to the shock phase in acute inflammation. An indication of a rudimentary antishock phase was only found ocassionally in early cases; generally, an MS exacerbation takes its course under the humoral picture of a pure shock phase. The parameter variations were, however, rather less (maximum of 25% in the electrolytes), and the course was significantly longer than in acute inflammation (by at leat 40–50 days = 6–7 weeks). There was no significant change in the parameters in the chronic-progressive form, particularly in the electrolytes – they mainly lay within the reaction level found in the shock phase of the acute and exudative-exacerbative type of reaction.

The three most important types of reaction were thus found – and they are still so today (see Fig. 8): the normal reaction form (RF), the RF of the exudative exacerbation and the RF of the chronic-progressive inflammations (*Perger* 1956). From 1954 it was possible to extend these longitudinal section hemograms in MS and acute febrile infections to internal chronic diseaes. Here, individual transitional forms from the normal to the morbid RF were found.

In particular the fourth important RF was found, that of the exacerbative, proliferative-degenerative RF, that runs into an antishock phase. These exacerbations are characterized by a particularly long course; the stage that has long been followed-up humorally lasts 231 days (= 33 weeks). This RF narrowly approaches blockade of ground regulation.

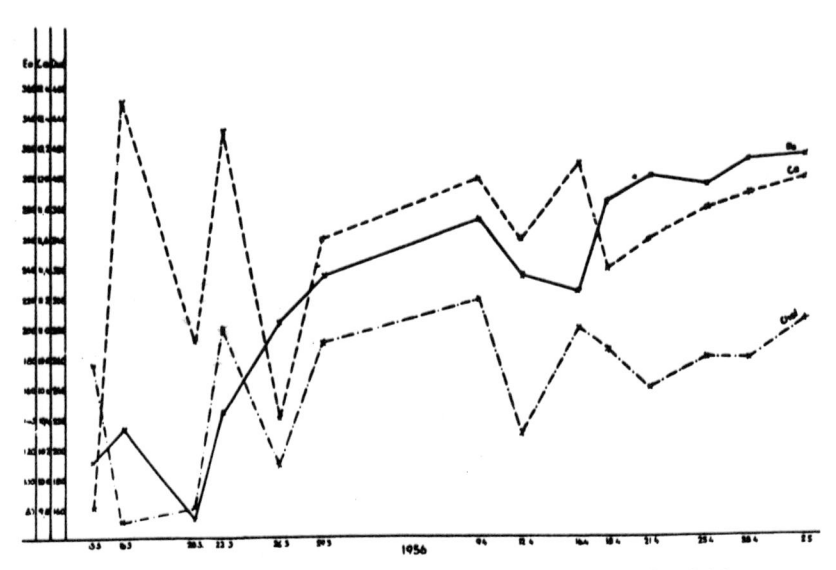

Fig. 7: Change from "atactic" to chronic reaction type in an untreated polyarthritis case, a 20 year old woman (from *F. Perger*, Ther. Wo. 8 [1958], 224)

It was possible to confirm the findings with serum electrophoresis: the progress of the globulin alterations is totally tied to the nonspecific RF. In particular, the development of γ-globulin elevation (IgA, IgM and IgG) depends on the process of nonspecific regulation; its maximum always lies at the end of the nonspecific inflammatory reactions, i.e. in the acute disease after 7–8 weeks, in exacerbations with an exudative character after 6–8 weeks, and in those with a proliferative-degerative character only after 25–35 weeks.

Anaphylactic reaction
(500–1.000 M/Vacc.)

Type: chronic progressive inflammation and in malignancy
(rehabilitation boundary cannot be established with vaccine)

Type: recurrent inflammation of exudative character
(1.000–20.000 M/Vacc.)

Type: recurrent inflammation of proliferative character
(500–10.000 M/Vacc.)

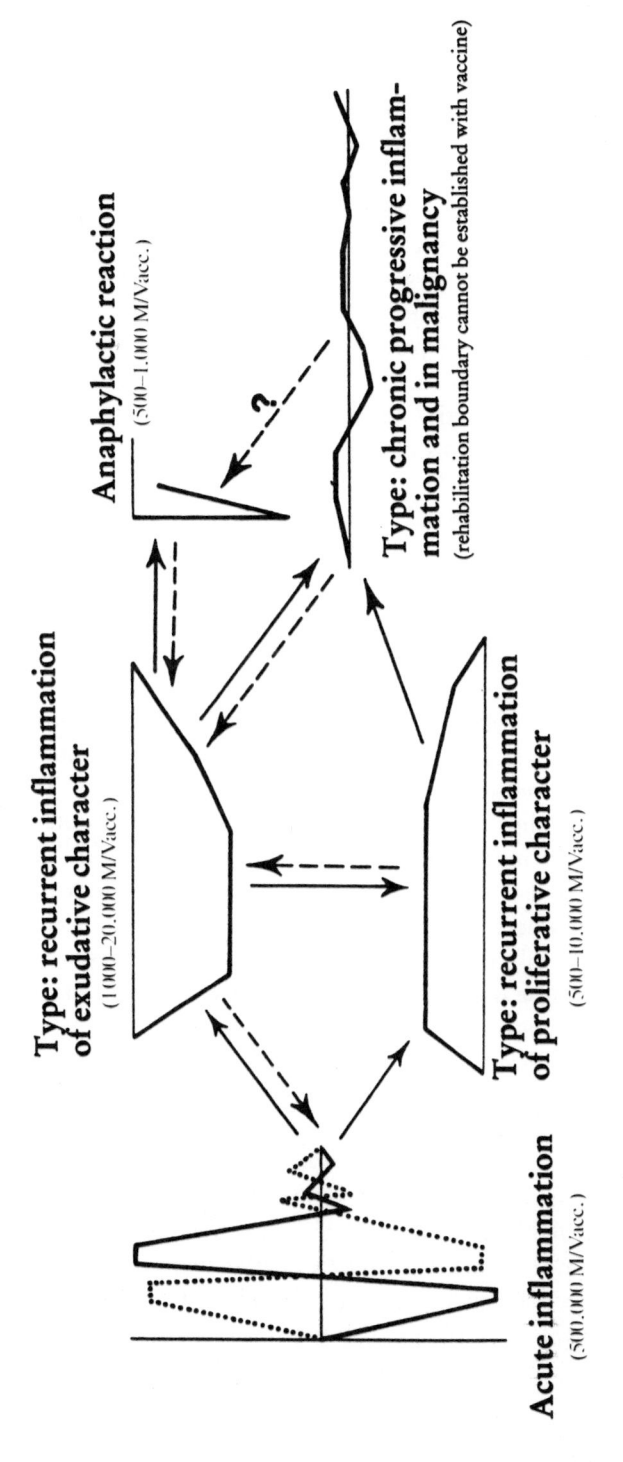

Acute inflammation
(500.000 M/Vacc.)

Fig. 8: Diagram of nonspecific reaction types according to *Perger*, corresponding to the similar calcium and cholesterin reactions, and, in regulatory disturbances, also of potassium. The figures in brackets indicate the vaccine quantity (M: microorganisms) that can initiate the reactions presented (from *F. Perger*, Phys. Med. u. Rehab. 20 [1979], 585).

This was the first indication that the speed and intensity of the specific immune reaction is closely coupled to ground regulation. This is a further indication that ground regulation is decisive and obiously contains or offers a system of order. In favour of this is the fact that pathological immunoglobins – e.g. the serum rheumatism samples – are sometimes also temporarily positive in the exacerbation forms, but only long-lasting when there is blockade of the ground functions and the course has a chronic-progressive character.

The nonreaction of the parameters of the nonspecific system had already been termed "blockade" by *Lutz* and *Pischinger* (1949), although the term was almost "paralysis". However, there is a clear difference between these two terms. Paralysis of nonspecific regulation can be temporary, and can also resolve itself spontaneously (e.g. after short-term chemotherapy), or can be resolved therapeutically (e.g. by neural therapy and acupuncture), but there are also paralyses of regulation that cannot be resolved (e.g. in PCP), and there is justification for calling these regulatory paralysis. Equally well, the regulatory paralysis in malignancies and the end-stages of chronic inflammations such as tuberculosis is true paralysis of function.

Regulatory blockade does not offer a standard picture like the other types of reaction, and an attempt has to be made to differentiate between resolvable and unresolvable blockade of the ground system. This is often successful from the specific clinical picture, but it can be decided from the level of the ICV in iodometry: greatly elevated ICVs with blockade are mainly resolvable – even if this is often difficult (ICV between 900 and 1,000 µg/ml); where the ICV is reduced they are no longer resolvable (ICV < 780 µg/ml). Evaluation of the resolvability of these "blockade" is important because the therapy concept is determined – rehabilitation of the defense functions or immunosuppressive therapy.

After clarification of these types of process on 4,716 patients and a minimum of 8 years of follow-up observation (*Perger* 1978) it was a logical step to determine how the patients react from the very beginning. An effective short-term test had to be developed for this.

Initially, this was tried with various types of vaccines, including autovaccines and heterovaccines. However, the results were completely different from the aim set. Instead of being able to establish the types of reaction in the vaccine test, the stimulus threshold for the totality reaction was found. True, this depended on the types of reaction in the longitudinal section hemogram, but it gave no information about the RF present.

The total of 917 tests with vaccines showed a pathophysiological phenomenon: up to a certain level, the periphery had an increasing inability to regulate and get over stimuli locally. In healthy subjects, the stimulus threshold is relatively high, at about 500,000 microorganisms per vaccine.

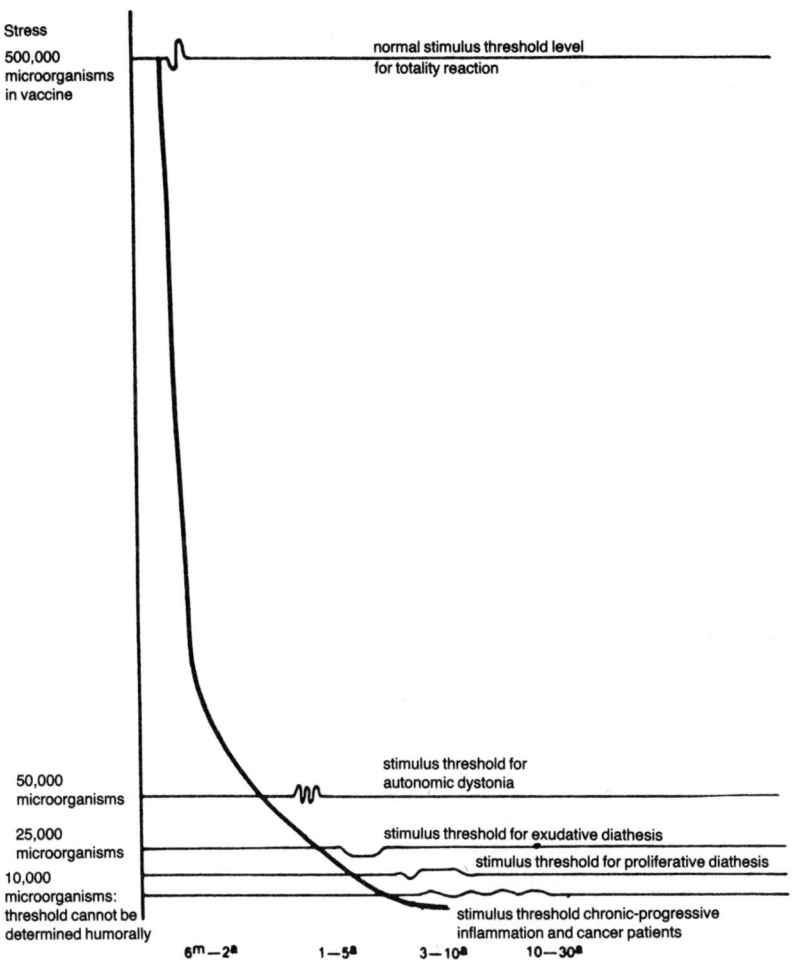

Fig. 9: Provisional diagram of stimulus thresholds for totality reactions in healthy subjects and patient with chronic-recurring and chronic-progressive diseases (from *F. Perger*, Entretiens de Monaco 1980, "Le rôle de la médecine moderne dans la crise du monde occidentale", p. 49-59, Clubs médecine informatique, Denisé, France, 1981).

However, in regulatory disturbances, it sinks rapidly, and finally sinks so low that it can no longer be measured by humoral testing methods. This means that the total defence of an organism has to be activated earlier and faster in chronic diseases, a completely uneconomical consumption of energy which leads in time to overconsumption (*Bergsmann* 1977).

The results of these stress test with vaccines had, however, clinical significance, since, for example, these reductions of the stimulus threshold are taken into account in desensitization therapy, and overreactions can be avoided; but the aim of obtaining a fast method of establishing the reaction type was not attained.

The solution to this question was brought by a clinical trial on the mechanism of action of monocyte factor, the triple-conjugated fatty acids, which was expanded by the available work already carried out by *Pischinger* (*Perger* 1956). As described in previous chapters, raising the amount of monocyte factor in the blood by injection produces a significant increase in the number of monocytes. However, this means a changeover from the microphage phase to the macrophage phase of cellular defense. This means that there is a simultaneous change from the humoral shock phase to the countershock phase, which also means a change from the prodromal phase to the active immunological phase. Humoral shock is resolved by the physiological increase and by the introduction of these particular fatty acids.

This special characteristic seemed to make the injection of this type of fatty acid suitable for bypassing the primary shock phase and obtaining the active defence processes of the countershock phase. This concept was successful.

After the first time blood was taken, factor M (ELPIMED®) was injected subcutaneously and the parameter changes after 1 and 4 hours were measured (later also after 3 hours) (*Perger* 1963).

It was already known from the longitudinal section hemograms that all regulatory disturbances can be diverted by *Selye's* alarm reaction. These deviations had already been started, but the following has to be mentioned: standstill in the shock phase (exudative-allergic-type processes), loss of the shock reaction and lapse into the countershock phase (proliferative-degenerative processes) and regulatory paralysis (blockade = chronic-progressive process, malignancies). In addition, the transitional forms from normal to pathological RF and the anaphylactic reaction, an acute, severe reaction within a few minutes.

Injection of factor M actually bypasses the shock phase, which is unavoidable with the injection of foreign substances. An organism shows its ability to process an immune-stimulating process within 3–4 hours.

Here, there are a variety of reaction forms (RF), which *Keller* (1979) has systematized on the basis of a statistical evaluation of 1,200 such tests.

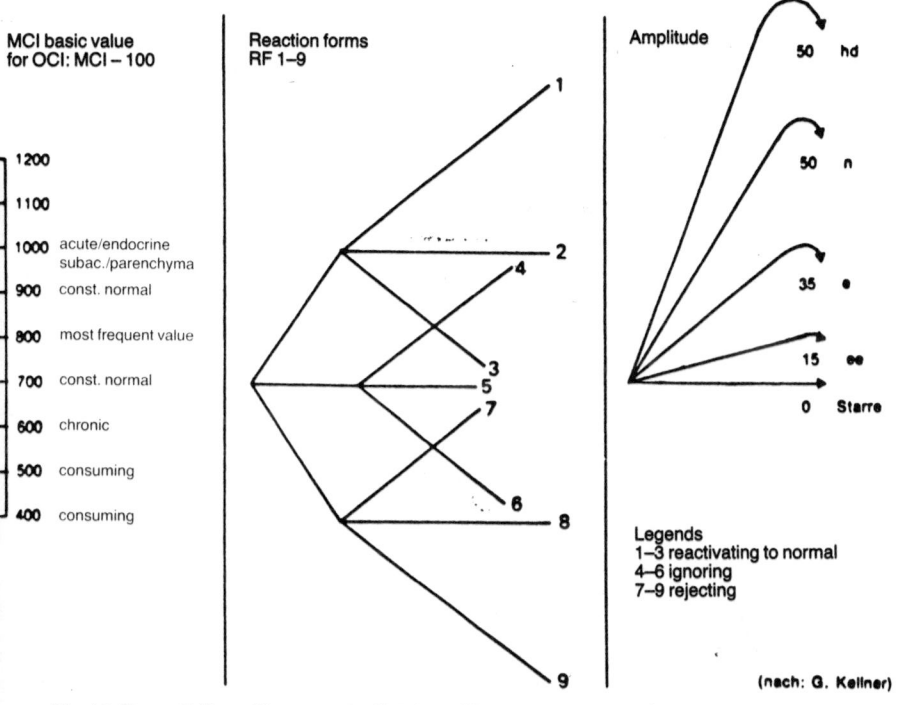

MCI basic value for OCI: MCI – 100		Reaction forms RF 1–9	Amplitude	
1200			50	hd
1100				
1000	acute/endocrine subac./parenchyma		50	n
900	const. normal		35	•
800	most frequent value			
700	const. normal		15	••
600	chronic		0	Starre
500	consuming			
400	consuming			

Legends
1–3 reactivating to normal
4–6 ignoring
7–9 rejecting

(nach: G. Kellner)

Fig. 10: From *Kellner, Krammer, Seidl,* Die Heilkunst 91 (1978), Heft 3.

Also, a healthy organism can regulate and recover from a moderate stimulus within 3–4 hours (RF 3). Simple blockade of the ground functions, e.g. after a simple common cold, after chemotherapy and with the initial, fleeting manifestations of an inflammatory systemic disease, lead to stronger and longer-lasting ICV reactions as a sign of greater activation of the defense system. In delayed convalsescence from a cold, a febrile exacerbation can sometimes be triggered, and the remnant of the infection is overcome. However, improvements in autonomic breakdowns and manifestations of systemic inflammation only appear temporarily, as the causes of these processes cannot be overcome by factor M (silent, chronic inflammations, scar disturbance fields, subclinical toxicosis, etc.). Care is needed in allergic diseases such as bronchial asthma. It is certainly unusual, but both *Pischinger* and the author of this chapter have triggered attacks of bronchial asthma with the injection – in my own two cases the cause was bacterial allergy. These reactions embrace RF-1 with excessive and long-lasting elevation of the ICV.

However, delayed allergy-type diseases that are already manifest (inflammatory forms of articular rheumatism, multiple sclerosis, ulcerative colitis, etc.) react after an hour, with intensification of the humoral shock phase (RF 7–9). This contradicted the finding that factor M is a host antishock substance. The question could be solved: with blood removal 30 minutes after the injection, a shock-triggering effect of these special fatty acids could be established.

The shock reaction only appeared after these 30 minutes. This is confirmation of the open, highly intermeshed system, described in the previous chapter. When the noxious factors causing the disease cannot be overcome there is *active* hindrance of the activation of immunological functions. This occurs in the central efforts of an open energy system, such as the human organism, to maintain life and avoid major damage. If an organism assesses activation of the immune processes as dangerous, it uses every opportunity to neutralize the activation. These processes require a large energy expenditure. This aspect has to be given serious consideration in chronic diseases.

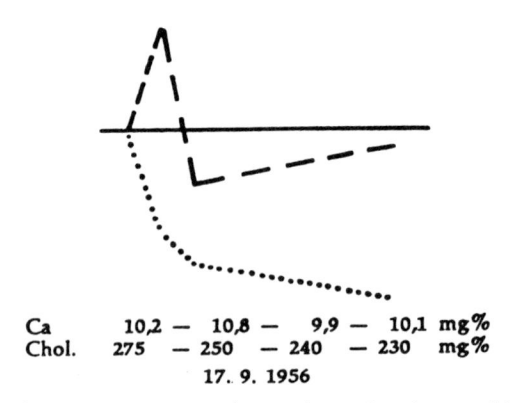

Ca	10,2 —	10,8 —	9,9 —	10,1	mg%
Chol.	275 —	250 —	240 —	230	mg%

17. 9. 1956

Fig. 11: Accelerated reaction process: even after 30 minutes the primary antishock reaction can be also measured by blood controls (from *F. Perger*, Oest. Z. f. Stomat. 60 [1963] 440).

This also makes it understandable why there is an absence of reaction in all the parameters of the immune system after a stimulus. Regulatory blockade, in *Kellner's* scheme RF 1–4, does not only affect the ICV; it also affects the electrolytes, deviations in the lipids, etc. Here, it has to be pointed out that, for example, the electrolytes indicate blockade much earlier than the ICV and oxymetry. All these are signs of energy exhaustion in the ground system, although this is not complete; very severe reactions continue to be blocked so far as possible. The chronic-progressive course of inflammatory diseases shows that this is no longer fully possible. Complete energy exhaustion is only seen shortly before death, as in the cavernous stage of phthisis, where a normalization of all parameters is found a few days before death. In any case, the exhaustion is so great that the slight stimulus by the test substance produces no reaction.

These tests were finally published (*Perger* 1969), based on 435 tests with ELPIMED alone, and a further 69 in combination with other substances. This had scarcely been published when *Bergsmann* (1965) reported on the asymmetry of autonomically-controlled factors. First of all he established significant differences between the leukocyte counts in the two halves of the body in unilateral tuberculous processes, and later also in unilateral focal stress. He assumed that the basis of this asymmetry was a side-difference in the perfusion of the vascular bed, possibly in the functioning of the arteriovenous anastomoses. This statement was, and is, doubted. The counter argument, which can still be heard today when physicians are confronted with the question for the first time, was that blood mixes itself continuously in the heart, and that differing values could therefore not exist. However, this argument only holds good for the arterial limb of the vascular system, and not for the path through the peripheral capillaries into the venous blood. Locally, tissue accepts the arterial blood offer, and surrenders what it can and must surrender.

With *Kellner, Pischinger* (1975) not only confirmed all the findings made by *Bergsmann* (1965) he expanded them with the fact that they could be demonstrated in the leukocyte count and all the other parameters of nonspecific regulation.

These side-differences were observed most clearly in the iodometry ICV and in oxymetry of venous blood; they were also found in the electrolytes, blood fats (total cholesterol), and finally they were also demonstrated in immunoglobulins A, M and G.

30 years earlier, a higher antibody titer had already been observed in unilateral inflammatory processes (*McMaster* and *Hudack* 1935), but attracted little notice. This earlier observation only gained significance in connection with ground system research, since this local increase in antibodies could be demonstrated as being functionally dependent on ground regulation.

Table 4 and Figures 12A and 12B show that there are various initial states and types of reaction in both sides of the body in many chronically ill patients. This can be seen even more clearly in the curves showing the progress.

In the course of the investigations it became more and more clear that the ground system reacted as an entirety, but not necessarily uniformly. The differences are the greater the less time a chronic disease has progressed. In the field of ground regulation, the time factor, the duration of the stress, plays an extremely important role in the extension of disturbances over the entire organism, and this will be examined in more detail later.

However, it is also clear from the asymmetry that a major amount of local autonomy has to be granted to the ground system, as could be seen from stimulation threshold determination. The oxyhemoglobin content of the arteries is equally high on both sides, lying between 96% and 98%. The first research on arterial oxyhemoglobin (femoral artery) and venous hemoglobin

Tab. 4

Prot. No.	Time in hours	% Oxy-Hb right / left	Jod VW in mg% right / left
65	0	55 / 48	103.9 / 103.4
	1	36 / 33	103.2 / 103.2
	3	38 / 46	100.2 / 98.2
66	0	50 / 60	90.7 / 89.2
	1	74 / 84	90.7 / 86.6
	3	87 / 90	90.7 / 89.6
71	0	66 / 83	100.7 / 97.5
	1	66 / 80	93.3 / 95.7
	3	51 / 60	94.0 / 91.2
77	0	64 / 44	82.4 / 77.9
	1	50 / 55	79.1 / 79.8
	3	64 / 56	84.3 / 79.1
83	0	42 / 22	90.6 / 01.0
			87.0 / 85.8
	1	38 / 27	87.4 / 86.2
		36 / 27	

REFLEX OXYMETRY Prot. Nr. 680314 plo-27

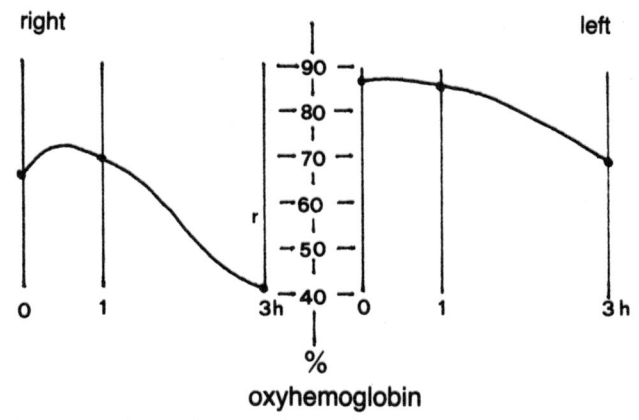

Fig. 12A: Differences in the initial value and type of reaction in oxymetry of venous blood (from the slide collection of Prof. G. *Kellner*, Histol.-Embryol. Institut, Vienna University).

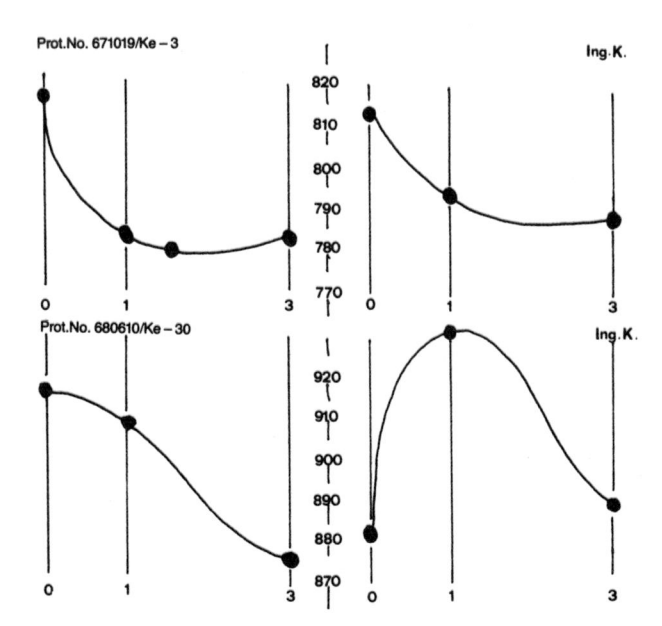

Fig. 12B: Differences in initial value and type of reaction in iodometry (from the slide collection of Prof. G. *Kellner*, Histol.-Embryol. Institut, Vienna University).

(cubital vein) was carried out by *Pischinger* and *Stacher* (*Pischinger* 1975), and showed this congruence of oxyhemoglobin in the arteries and the side-different values in venous blood. This has been confirmed in trials by other investigators, in both hemoglobin and electrolyte determinations (Ca, K, Mg).

Response to the question of whether these processes are under central regulation or more from peripheral autonomy comes out more in favour of peripheral autonomy. This opinion is also supported by the fact that the more seriously disturbed initial state and type of reaction are both found in the more severely stressed side. It is always a matter of an unavoidable tissue disintegration which is found to be the cause of such side differences. At the same time, it is irrelevant whether it is a matter of inflammatory disturbances (so-called foci), inorganic stress (e.g. operation scars with talcum crystal inclusions, war wounds with shrapnel and the remnants of material or accident scars containing sand, asphalt, or glass splinters). Moreover, two furhter investigations have to be taken into consideration that give greater significance to peripheral disturbances than central control. Both investigations concern cell cultures that permitted observation of functions, without central nervous or hormonal influences.

Kellner (1963) showed that the acid-base balance is regulated in the ground system; in an acid medium the pH value is restored to neutral by breakdown of fibroblasts; in an alkaline medium it is restored by fibroblast proliferation. In the same year, *McLaughlin* (1963) published his findings on embryonic epidermal cell cultures. In vitro, embryonic epidermal cells proliferate in a completely haphazard and undifferentiated way; they only differentiate when mesenchymal cells are added, forming a basement membrane, and then grow in orderly layers. With two completely different targets and methods, these two experiments show that there is a system of order in the ground tissue, and that it is independent of central influences. For all these reasons, the side-differences, the level of the threshold stimulus, the localization of the stress, and the cell cultures, it can be assumed that there really is ground system autonomy.

However, the existence of functional autonomy does not mean that this cannot be influenced by other systems. The opposite is the case: the intermeshing of the regulatory systems is so intensive that no decision can be made in healthy subjects as to which regulatory system actually controls the nonspecific functions. Hence, one can say that physiology has also passed by the insignificant extracellular matrix; the lymph nodes and hormonal glands and the CNS are far more imposing organs, beside which the extracellular substance is a diffuse, difficult to grasp and hardly recognizable organ system. It is only possible to recognize the activity of the individual systems in disturbances of the defense mechanism when their absence of activity becomes apparent.

Even then a clear classification is not always possible. This can be seen in the measurements of electrical phenomena and skin temperature (R and C measurements according to *Kracmar* [1961]), decoder impulse dermography or thermoregulatory measurements according to *Schwamm* (1955): with these regulatory disturbances, who can make a clear decision on whether peripheral autonomy or central control predominates? Naturally, there is a tendency, based on experiences with humoral parameters, to estimate the role of the periphery in electrical and thermal regulatory disturbances relatively highly. In addition, there are observations: in early cases, both measurements show disturbances in the area of the affected segments; rather later in the course, the disturbances attack the homolateral half of the body, and a disturbance of the electrical and thermal reactions of the entire organism can only be shown in the late stages. However, even then the affected segment still shows the high intensity of these disturbances. The extension of these changes over the site without participation of the autonomic nerve centers can scarcely be imagined. The intensive intermeshing of the regulatory system cannot be simply and suddenly denied where it creates special reasoning difficulties.

The question here is how and via which routes (=regulatory system) the disturbance can spread itself over the field of a local disintegration. It must be remembered that every "focus" and every "disturbance field" reaches into the connective tissue as the bearer of nonspecific regulation (*Pischinger* 1954, 1956). According to *Pischinger*, the spread of local regulatory disturbance can take place reflexly over the communication routes of the ground system, particularly via a bilateral structure that, without curtailing the totality of the ground system structure, means a certain amount of independence in the two halves of the body. This possibility is offered only by the nervous system with its graduated structure from its synaptic terrain to the brain field via the brain stem and midbrain.

A thought should be added to these considerations by *Pischinger*. It is of course only a hypothesis, but nevertheless worth closer investigation. It is known that tissue disintegrations – whether of organic or inorganic nature – produce an acidosis in the milieu at the site in question. However, as *Pischinger* (1954, 1956) and *Kellner* (1963) have shown, acidosis leads on the one hand to release of fibroblasts from their cellular contacts into free blood cell forms (large reticular cells: monocytes, histiocytes, small reticular cells: lymphocytes), and on the other hand to their breakdown to regulate the tissue milieu back to a neutral pH value. Since, however, as *Heine* (personal information) reported, no significant fibroblast deficiency is found in chronic inflammatory foci as compared to the wider surroundings, these local, continuing losses must be replaced from the environment. This is conceivable for the local area, and could also be the case for the segmental area. One therefore has to determine the fibroblast density in the local and segmental area, as well as in distant, undisturbed segments. This would also be important for the explanation and acceptance of the effects of the so-called foci. For the focus – the silent, chronic inflammation – only has a direct-causal connection with the secondary disease in a very low percentage of the affected patients, and is only a predisposing factor for the inflammatory systemic disease, as already classified by *Kerl* (1932) and *Urbach* (1935) (*Perger* 1978).

During further investigation, stresses from toxic heavy metals and deficiency states were recorded. The toxin stress concerned the heavy metals lead, cadmium and mercury, and to some extent nickel. The degree of stress was still subsymptomatic, i.e. there were no clear symptoms of chronic poisoning – for this reason the definition is subsymptomatic toxicosis. However, even subsymptomatic stresses can lead to defence disturbances in their depots, although these have less effect on the ground system and more on the enzymatic processes in immunoglobulin formation. At the same time deficiencies in the Coferment-heavy metals (iron, copper, zinc, selenium and manganese) and in minerals (calcium, potassium and magnesium) were recorded. However, it is outside the reference of this book to give all the details of these research results.

It is particularly interesting that only minimal, and sometimes no side differences appeared with immune stimulation (in the ELPIMED test) in focal and disturbance field processes. The toxicoses and deficiency states have a diffuse effect, and give evidence of the particularities of local tissue changes through silent, chronic inflammation and scar disturbance fields.

This is a remarkable difference in nonspecific regulatory behaviour and has an important therapeutic consequence: operative removal of foci and disturbance fields without paying attention to the toxic stresses and deficiency states can result in complete failure of the therapy concept. Here, zinc deficiency has the greatest significance. For this means that the toxic heavy metals cannot be washed out, and therefore block a variety of enzymatic reactions in their depots. In deficiency states it also means that other enzymatic activities can also be inactivated. The enzyme metallothionine is responsible for the chelating and washing out of toxic heavy metals, but needs zinc as a co-ferment for its activity, and zinc is also needed for DNA and RNA polymerase activity; a disturbance of the RNA polymerases also leads to limitation of immunoglobulin synthesis, which can lead in turn to a deficiency of urgently necessary IgG (*Perger* 1986, 1987). The residual focal formation after operative processes (e.g. tonsillar scar abscesses, etc.) are a common consequence of zinc deficiency, since immune reactions such as T-cell activation and IgG synthesis are delayed and inadequate. The development of these zinc deficiency states and of other trace elements has been recorded since 1980, and shows a rising tendency (*Perger* 1987).

A further fact has not yet been explained: the behaviour of the trace elements (Fe, Cu, Zn) is generally extremely stable in the immune stimulation test. Certainly, minimal variations do occur, particularly in allergic reaction types. With ELPIMED as test stimulus, the total serum protein

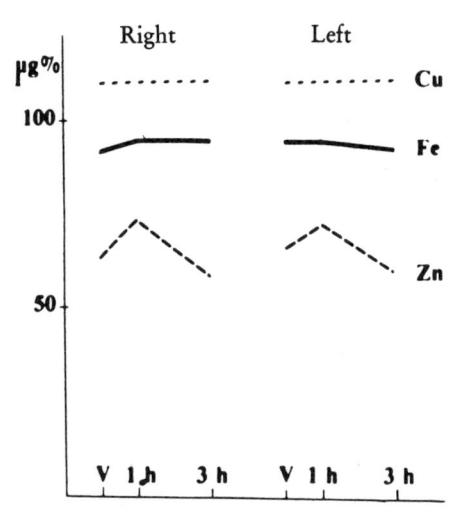

Fig. 13A: Stable behaviour of trace elements inter test stimulus: seronegative oligoarthritis.

content often sinks by 0.2–0.4% within the first hour – the minimal variations of the trace elements are clearly related to this dilution effet. However, in greatly advanced chronic-progressive inflammation, a high Fe and Cu lability, and particularly of Zn is sometimes found, which greatly exceeds the dilution effect.

Up to now, the reason for this has not been clearly defined. It is, however, a fact that it is only found in cases of complete paralysis of the ground system, with a raised and disordered readiness of the immune system to react. One can thus label the cause as a complete dissociation between the ground system and the immune system. The difference between complete paralysis of the ground system and the over-reaction of the immune system is astonishing. In the most extreme case observed, the IgG rose by 1466 mg% within three hours, and also led to a stronger reaction in an existing primary-chronic polyarthritis (it was possible to cushion this reaction with ACTH).

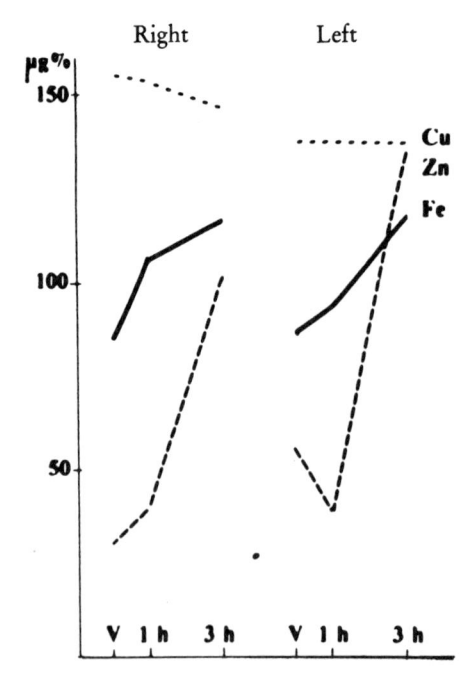

(Fig. 13B: Labile behaviour of trace elements under test stimulus: advanced seropositive PcP. (Figs. 13 from F. *Perger*, Oest. Z. f. Stomat. 80 [1983] 289).

A complete dissociation between the ground and immune system can be assumed in lability of the trace elements; rehabilitation of the function of both systems was not possible in any of these cases, and in addition to this, there is extensive exhaustion of the hypophyseal-adrenal function in all these cases. Nevertheless, the patients can be helped by the usual immune suppression methods. From this, it can be seen that the inclusion of ground regulation in the diagnostic procedure makes it possible to determine whether rehabilitation of the defense functions is still possible or not, and that it can provide a sensible adjunct to the two therapeutic concepts of immune rehabilitation and immune suppression.

Determination of the types of reaction and the various stresses shows yet another detail that has to be emphasized. The ground system has a nonspecific but constant reaction to all types of stimulus. For this reason, these varying stimuli have an accumulative effect: it is constantly shown that the individual qualities of the stimuli are too weak to bring about disturbances of function in the nonspecific system on their own; but together they cause the pathological stimulus response. This was obvious in patients where the stresses took place due to several simultaneous chronic inflammations, from toxicoses and intestinal flora aberrations.

This additive effect is one of the most important results of ground system research. It also depends on the time factor, the duration of the various stresses.

It is therefore necessary to recognize certain facts:
1. The ground system reacts as a totality, but not necessarily uniformly,
2. Reaction differences depend on the sites of the stresses (bacterial and non-bacterial tissue disintegration),
3. The ground system has a certain amount of peripheral autonomy, but this can be lost at an early stage in chronic inflammation,
4. Since it reacts in a completely unspecific way, a great variety of stimuli and stresses can accumulate, and derail its functions; summation effect (chronic inflammation, toxins, deficiencies, intestinal flora aberration),
5. It reacts according to *Selye's* alarm reaction, and its disturbances are derived from this,
6. Dissociation of the normal intermeshing of the ground regulation system and the immune regulation system (always combined with exhaustion of pituitary-adrenal function) cannot be restored to normal with the means available today.

Extraneural Mechanism for Control of Defence Processes

Four cellular phases are known in defence processes.

First of all the histiocyte wall forms around the invasion site of a noxious agent; the microphage phase takes place immediately after this – also still local, but as if with a more passive accompanying reaction by the entire organism. Next comes the third phase, the macrophage phase, and this is accompanied by full active participation of the entire organism, the fourth phase is the lymphocyte phase (with overcoming or chronification of an infection).

With discovery of monocyte factor and the clarification of its position in the defence processes it became more and more clear that this M factor is important for actuating the macrophage phase. The consequence of deficiency of triple-conjugated fatty acids or their inactivity (high, but fixed values in the regulation test) is that the macrophage phase is too small or cannot be measured at all. This means that its function does not come about.

However, this question does not mean that central nervous regulations have to be denied. They are part of an extraneural milieu that, together with central control, is important for defence processes. The question, precisely formulated, is: apart from monocyte factor, are there other humoral substances that are also decisive for actuating the various cellular phases, and which factors outside neural control are also of importance if no humoral substances come into the question?

It is typical of a completely new research field, such as the ground system, that these thought processes only come into the foreground at a relatively late stage. One picks ones way through a labyrinth and has to feel the way forward step by step, based on the available facts. Ground system research began with the fact of the discovery of monocyte factor with its completely unspecific reactions. Explanation of its effects needed explanation of the histological structure of the intercellular substance and finally took the various reactions after injection of this factor into account, and the asymmetry of the reactions in the two halves of the body complicated this research even more. Parallel to this, recognition and evaluation of the causes of defence disturbances in the nonspecific system and the significance of the asymmetries was a full-time affair. Nevertheless, *Pischinger* had already started to look for further humoral factors that might play a role in the defence function processes in 1967. In 1975 – at the time the first edition of this book was published – these efforts had not yet been rewarded with success.

Pischinger was only able to report the discovery of a second substance that played a role in the cellular process four years later, in 1975.

The current state of knowledge of the actuation of the various cellular phases is given in sequence below.

The first local defence processes are initiated by a series of tissue hormones (prostaglandins, leukotriens, interferons, etc.). However, the histiocyte wall and microphage phases are activated by both biochemical and biophysical processes, e.g. through the abrupt change in the pH value at the invasion site of a noxious agent – through acidosis and the resulting changes in the cell membranes. As already described (*Perger* 1984), this – seen biologically – is really very logical. A humoral process or a biochemical reaction always needs a certain amount of time to create an adequate concentration to have an effect. This would be a dangerous loss of time for the organism. The abrupt change in the biophysical situation at the invasion site leads to a so-called emergency reaction – it initiates the first defence reactions at once, which are predominantly containment measures. These are summarized in two phases.

1. Release of large reticular cells from their local bindings in the ground system; as free cells these form a wall around the invasion site, as mononuclear histiocytes.
2. Changes in the permeability of the capillary walls, followed by the microphage phase.

The microphage phase is not limited to migration of granulocytes to the invasion site. The granulocytes phagocytose invading microorganisms and partly break down under the release of oxidative and proteolytic agents, and thus fight the invasion locally. At the same time local edema develops due to the transfer of blood serum into the tissue. This has two effects: the edema leads to further dilution of the noxious agent, and immunoglobulins already available from previous infections can be effective immediately at the invasion site. The significance of local edema was subject to controversy for some time, for some researchers saw a danger of microorganisms being carried from the locality into the entire organism, but finally it was recognized that this dilution opposed a "high zone" paralysis, an inhibition of defense due to too high concentrations of microorganisms or toxins (*Humphrey* and *Withe* 1972). A hypothetical consideration can also be brought up. Energy reactions can also be initiated by the change in the pH. It should not be forgotten that every active process also needs energy. The necessary AT-phosphatases have to be activated. On the one hand, this depends on an adequate concentration of calcium in the extracellular tissue fluid and the calcium-magnesium relationship in this energy system; on the other – so far as can be said from the available information – on the intensity of the pH alteration. A tissue that is already acidotic (e.g. in diabetes and/or silent chronic inflammation, false nutrition, etc.) only shows a relatively minor pH change, so this minor increase in acidosis has an equally minor influence on the total reaction, including energy release.

All experience indicates that this start-energy has major, and even decisive importance for the further course of an illness. In every noxious agent invasion process a start-energy deficiency can hardly ever be made good the the further course of a disease. This also underlines the importance of ground regulation.

So much for the known and supposed processes for activating the first two local cellular reactions.

Central nervous and organic reactions (CNS, hormone system, lymph nodes), as well as humoral substances needed for the activation of the macrophage and lymphocyte phases are responsible for the following phases.

Activation of the macrophage phase with all its accompanying reactions is a main theme of this book and was described in detail by *Pischinger* (1975). The humoral-autonomic shock phase, monocytosis and activation of the entire defence system (change to the humoral antishock phase = start of the acute phase) in the contest between the healthy organism and the invading noxious agent only takes place with the active participation of monocyte factor, which depends on its propagation in the intercellular substance and the serum.

The increase in the concentration of this factor in the extracellular matrix is decisive. This is easily demonstrated by the various types of monocyte factor (ELPIMED®). The greatest systemic effect follows subcutaneous injection, as a rich supply of soft connective tissue is present there. Intramuscular injection also meets extracellular substance, and hardly any lessening of the effect can be recognized. A systemic effect can hardly ever be established with intravenous injection and this can be seen to depend on dilution in the blood. Intradermal injection, as described by *Busch* and *Busch* (1978) certainly has a strong local effect, but there is very little systemic reaction. Oral dosage is senseless as the fatty acid deriva-

tives are broken down – a normal HCl concentration in the stomach leads to hydrogenation of the unsaturated bindings, and part of the evidence of the effect of these bindings was the fact that no further biological effect could be actuated after hydrogenation of these bindings (*Pischinger*).
These effects are summarized below:
1. Initiation of humoral-autonomic shock states with a raised calcium concentration and reduced magnesium concentration in the tissue fluid.
2. Increase in the number of monocytes in the blood, and reduction of the lymphocytes.
3. Increased blood leukocytolysis rate.
4. Reduction of venous blood oxyhemoglobin as a sign of increased peripheral oxygen utilization.
5. Serum β and γ globulin fraction is changed and increased.

These reactions are obvious in healthy defence function, but gradually disappear in the course of regulatory system disturbances until they cannot be seen, and they can even be reversed.

The effect is thus particularly clear in delayed recovery after a banal common cold. Often, only one, sometimes 2–3 monocyte factor injections suffice to break down this defence inhibition. A transient fever appears in some patients. The reason for this blockade of defense is usually an attempt to suppress the cold for family or professional reasons. This is successful with the use of antipyretics, but only at the price of initiating a humoral shock reaction that persists for 2–4 months.

Similar shock reactions occur after skull injuries (contussion, cerebral contusion) and cerebaral insult. These shock states can also be resolved by monocyte factor. Obviously, destroyed cerebral tissue cannot be restored, but there is usally edema or ischemic zones around the affected area whose loss of function is still reversible. Redress of this "focal" reaction leads to rapid activation of the residual function. Naturally, the effect depends on the size of these zones, and at first this cannot be established clinically; for the reason, astonishingly large remissions are sometimes experienced; in other cases there is only minimal improvement. The effect of monocyte factor is greater than i.v. application of theophylline derivatives, and after more than 30 years of experience, is without the risk of causing secondary bleeding. Shock states after fractures, wounds and burns are also resolved rapidly, and specific necessary care can be initiated. This resolution of shock leads to the patient recovering more rapidly, and clearly accelerates the healing process.

All the examples given concern completed processes where there is no threat of activation of inflammation.

However, chemotherapeutics also belong to the humoral-autonomic shock theme. Most of the highly efficacious chemotherapeutics lead to such shock states as a side effect. They are often concerned with the known specific side effects.

Discovery of the alarm reaction in stress by *Selye* (1952) is also significant for chemotherapy, since every exogenous stimulus initiates – and this includes the use of therapeutic substances – this alarm reaction. In predamaged defense functions, however – apart from the intended specific effect – the undesired humoral stress reaction is activated and often responses with a derailment reaction, depending on the existing defense situation. The allergic reactions are based on the pathological stimulus response when an exudative shock reaction takes place. Toxic consequences are possible if there is blockade of the ground functions. Control of the nonspecific parameters on various highly efficacious chemotherapeutic substances has shown this.

The result is that combination of the leading antirheumatic drugs of the phenylbutazone range that have been on the market for three decades with monocyte factor (ELPIMED®) reduced the side effect rate to practically zero. The combination of antibiotic therapy with monocyte factor and intensification of the specific effect still has no side effects today (allergies, immune suppression, damage to the hemopoetic system). Failure of antibiotics that are effective in vitro but not in vivo can also be corrected by giving monocyte factor at the same time – the blockade of nonspecific regulation is prevented.

Two further observations have to be made since they give a confusing impression at first: if a corticoid is injected in combination with ELPIMED® the cortisone effect increases significantly, but if the factor is only injected 2–3 hours after the corticoid, the effect of the corticoid on the ground system is cancelled rapidly, i.e. a humoral shock (inhibitory) phase is seen again after another hour. A similar situation was observed with alcohol: the hangover after alcohol abuse is relieved by an ampoule of ELPIMED® in half an hour to an hour. However, if an attempt is made to avoid the hangover by injecting ELPIMED shortly before taking alcohol, one gets drunk faster – this undesired effect was observed in two colleagues from California in 1960; a quarter liter of wine after the "prophylactic" injection was enough of make them drunk, although they were both used to wine.

This is evidence of the intensification of the specific effect of this substance, which is explained by the actuation of the primary humoral shock phase.

During acute infections, the use of monocyte factor is therefore not indicated. Its use in chronic systemic diseases is more subtle. This activates the inflammatory processes, but care has to be taken that this activation is not too strong. One injection to test the defence situation is justifiable, but several doses cannot be justified without knowledge of the silent, chronic inflammation present. Here, activation of the local processes is possible and a reaction in the secondary localization is to be feared. Immune stimulation with the factor for example, permits recognition of scar abscesses after tonsillectomy, but the attempt to activate a secondary phenomenon with procaine or lidocaine as described by *Huneke* (1983) is preferable.

In after-treatment after elimination of the various stresses (foci, toxins, etc.) and after correction of deficiencies, the monocyte factor is once more of value, *Lutz* (1949) used alternating stimuli to activate the ground system: first of all he gave ELPIMED for 2–3 days, followed by an injection with 4–8 IE old insulin, to activate a nonspecific shock – repeated several times in succession. He was able to activate regulatory blockade with this "alternating therapy" (*Pischinger* 1975). This method of reactivating nonspecific functions has also proved its value in our own field, but it was given up due to the resulting weight increase from the small insulin shock, and the therapy described above preferred.

The ideal extension for activation of the defence regulatory system was then treatment with lymphocyte factor. After many years *Pischinger* (1979) finally found this factor in the venous lymph sinuses.

Factor "L" was found in lymph node extracts that were free of protein and triglycerides. This residual extract has an absorption maximum of 2,600 Å in the UV absorption spectrum. If other substances are added, the absorption curve shifts to 2,700 Å (*Pischinger* 1979). According to personal information from *Kellner*, these include ATP and Zn in particular.

The UV absorption maximum indicates that these substances are nucleotides – in normal serum the absorption maximum of uric acid is near this figure (2,900 Å). However, there is not yet enough clarity about these substances, and licensing as a drug is not possible at the moment.

In animal experiments (guinea pigs), the factor showed a major effect on the blood picture: lymphocytosis takes place, reaching its maximum after about 24 hours. The outpouring of lymphocytes from the lymph nodes is so great with high doses that an almost 100% emptying of the nodes was established in guinea pigs (*Pischinger* 1979). The emptying takes place in both the cortex and medulla – this confirms that both B and T lymphocytes are activated and move into the blood circulation. This point is extremely important for the starter function of this factor – cell-mediated and humoral lymphocyte reactions can be seen to begin at the same time and to the same degree.

At the same time as the lymphocytosis, a reduction of the blood monocytes begins, not percent but absolute. This is also typical of the normal (spontaneous) lymphocyte phase, and can be taken as evidence that this lymph extract really is the humoral substance for actuating this cellular defence phase.

Pischinger (1983) describes the lymphocyte increase in animal experiments as being from 28.7 plus or minus 5.4% to 70.2 plus or minus 7.8%, and in a second trial from 49.9 plus or minus 12% to 68.6 plus or minus 11% within 24 hours after subcutaneous injection of the extract. At the same time, the monocyte count regresses from 2.4% to 1.1%.

Pischinger and the author of this chapter first of all carried out several trials on themselves to clarify the question of the applicability of the extract for human beings. The lymph extract was only used on other people after this. The lymphocytosis appeared in humans, as in guinea pigs, but the peak value appeared much sooner, after 3 hours. The reaction was regressing after 24 hours in all the test subjects.

The extent of the lymphocytic reaction depends on the dose and the individual defence state of the test subject. In disturbed host defense, the reaction is often lower or significantly higher than in healthy subjects, but after several injections it approaches the normal level. The increase in lymphocytes in the differential blood picture was noticeable, particularly in older people: the greatest increase was found in a 74 year old after injecting 1 ml of the extract with a dry content of 0.5%: the lymphocytes increased from 21% to 64%, i.e. they increased by a factor of three within 3 hours.

This reaction is accompanied by an increase in γ-globulins, which can be shown after 3 hours, but the peak value is only reached after 24–48 hours. With starch gel thin-layer electrophoresis according to *Maruna* and *Gründig* (1968), it could be shown that the increase is mainly in the IgG, while the IgM level sinks both actually and as a percentage. A few other investigations, which could not be followed up for external reasons, indicated that the T cell population is also stimulated.

Higher concentrations (1.0–1.2% dry substance/ml) often led to acute activation of chronic inflammation, with the appearance of fever. For this reason, dilutions with a dry content of 0.5% and later 0.1–0.2% were produced. With a dry substance of 0.2% it was then possible to control the lymphocyte reaction in such a way that no general reaction or fever were activated, with doses rising from an initial 0.2–0.3 ml once to twice weekly, and the clinical effect was obtained.

However, in severe inflammatory systemic diseases, using solutions with 0.2% dry substance/ml showed a rather protracted immunoglobulin reaction in comparison to that from using the initial concentrations of 1.0% or 0.5%.

The reaction was, of course, weaker in the more banal chronic types of inflammation, such as chronic bronchitis, but regular. However, there were significant differences within the first hours after the injection in patients with multiple sclerosis or inflammatory rheumatism of the joints.

Tumor patients react rather differently.

a) Inflammatory forms of joint rheumatism.

In 24 patients with seronegative and seropositive polyarthritis, injection of 0.3 ml of a 0.2% solution of the lymph extract was followed by a reduction of IgA and IgM of between 8% and 17% within three hours, and initially, IgG also regressed by an average of 5–7%. After 24 hours there was an isolated elevation of IgG of 13% above the initial value, on average. The initial reduction in serum immunoglobulins is scarcely a breakdown, rather a transfer into the tissues; the later increase in IgG can also be connected with an increased leukolysis rate.

b) Multiple sclerosis

In 22 multiple sclerosis patients, the IgG rose by 10–15% in the first three hours, the IgM by about 4–5%, just above the error limits of the study, and IgG sank by about 10%. There was a slight increase in IgG after 24 hours, but this averaged only 4%. This slight reaction indicates a severe disturbance of the humoral immune reaction in MS,

c) Malignant tumors

In 55 tumor patients – all after operation on the primary tumor – a drop in IgM of about 13% was observed within 3 hours; IgA and IgG rose at the same time by about 5%, and by about a further 8% after 24 hours.

These reactions in all three patient groups also depend on zinc content, in particular: with a serum zinc of less than 30 µg/dl, these immunoglobulin changes cannot be initiated. The lymph extract is also unable to activate the RNA polymerases, as these need zinc as a coenzyme for ribonucleic acid synthesis. Whether, and to what extent zinc deficiency has an adverse effect on leukolysis has not yet been investigated.

But a raised specific antibody titer was also observed. From 1983, due to the theory of slow-virus genesis of MS, the AB titer against rubella, measles, Eppstein-Barr virus and toxoplasmosis was determined. It stands out that there were slight increases in AB titer against 2 or 3 of this series, with only a few exceptions. The titers were 1:32 and 1:64 even when these infections had taken place years before – in healthy people these AB titers were only 1:8 or 1:16. With very careful use of the lymph extract (0,1 ml of the 0.1% solution as initial dose with a gradual increase to 0.1 ml once weekly) the AB titers rise slowly to 1:512 and then return to the normal level of 1:16. There is stabilization of the clinical course at the same time. This provides additional confirmation of the viral genesis of multiple sclerosis – but it also shows that there have usually been several viral stresses, and in some cases also toxoplasmosis. If this should be confirmed by further investigation, it would be an important step in explaining the etiology of this disease.

The AB-increasing effect of lymph extract was also confirmed in rheumatism patients: in patients with silent chronic inflammation (foci), the ASLO titer rose to 2,000 IV.

The effect of lymph extract on the B lymphocytes can be seen clearly from these results.

However, the effect on the T lymphocytes has to be further investigated. In our investigations this was not possible for external reasons. Nevertheless, some information can be given.

In a 45 year old patient with breast cancer, the T lymphocyte activity was checked preoperatively, at another site. The findings indicated full inactivity of this cell population. After 10 injections of increasing doses of a 0.1% solution, control showed that all sub-groups of T lymphocytes were reactivated, although not completely.

It is not possible, however to bring about complete tumor regression. This could be measured at two local breast cancer recurrences during the preoperative preparation time: the tumors regressed, but did not disappear. In an operated seminoma with abdominal lymph node invasion and a large metastasis in the left kidney, the lymph node metastases regressed so much that the surgeon could find no indication of lymph node invasion during the kidney metastasis operation – but the kidney metastasis had not been affected by the lymph extract.

In these 3 patients, a lack of lymph extract led to rapid recurrence of the tumors, so rapidly that 2 of the patients died after a short time. Experience with 15 other tumor patients indicates that a certain group of patients need the lymph extract life-long – rather like a diabetic needing insulin. There is every indication that patients with an iodine utilization of less than 780 µg/dl are no longer able to synthesise the lymphocyte factor. On the other hand, another group of postoperative tumor patients is able to do this: those with a high IUV (850–1000 µg/ml), who are not able to react. If the reaction capacity of the unsaturated bindings can be restored – and the lymph extract is extremely suitable for this, although other methods also seem to be possible, e.g. mistletoe preparations – long-term therapy is not needed. These observations were first made on a colleague with 3 primary tumors (1. bladder papilloma, 2. seminoma 10 years later, 3. larynx carcinoma 2 years later); 5 years after host defense activation he had no manifestations of malignancy, but unfortunately died in an accident.

The effect on the T lymphocyte population was probably made more obvious by the effects in intestinal mycoses. A high percentage of tumor patients suffer from mycoses of more than 10^6 fungi/g stool. Patients without tumors or late cases of chronic-progressive systemic inflammation with such quantities of fungi (Cand. alb. and spec., Trichosporum. spec., Rhodorulata spec., and Geotrichum spec. etc.) can be treated successfully as follows: first of all the patient receives the antimycotic that is most effective in vitro, for 10 days; then 3–4 months of milieu therapy with dextrorotatory lactic acid and freeze-dried symbiont. In this period the fungi are reduced to less than 10^2 or they are eliminated completely. However, this therapy does not work in tumor patients and those with late-stage, chronic-progressive inflammatory systemic disease. Supposedly, it is certain that fungal defense depends on the cell-mediated immune performance (T cells). Under therapy with the lymph extract, the intestinal mycoses disappear completely – without additional local therapy. As regards tumor therapy, the antimycotic effect of the extract also explains the influence on tumor growth – humoral performance fails due to the known enhancement effect. As shown from previous reports, previous experiences do not indicate that conservative therapy of malignancies is possible, since massive tumors cannot be made to regress. As before, operation, to reduce tumor load, is absolutely necessary. However, there are new aspects in postoperative defense stimulation treatment.

A surprising effect in schizophrenia was also observed. Patients who were about to be commited to mental hospitals due to the reappearance of hallucinations could be returned to normal society. The hallucinations disappeared. The mechanism of effect in this disease is, however, completely open, and the small number of patients does not permit the assumption of a definite effect in all types of schizophrenia. This aspect of the effects of lymph extract therefore needs further investigation. The effect on oxyhemoglobin and iodine utilization values is comparable to that of monocyte factor, but is – so far as can be established – not so strong. Here, however, there are no adequate results on healthy subjects, since the extract was only available in limited amounts. It is also highly regrettable that it has not been possible up to now to make at least small quantities available for further investigation; the investigations have had to be stopped since the spring of 1986.

However, these investigations show that using the two substances of the ground regulation system, monocyte factor and lymphocyte factor, it is possible to treat disturbances of the cellular and humoral immune processes at the right phase, and thus attack disease processes in a more physiological way than was possible in the past.

Neural Therapy According to Huneke

There are many causes of irritation of the ground system. So far as can be shown with the investigation methods available, there is *hardly any interference* with the organism that does not affect the nonspecific ground functions. This is shown by the puncture reaction. Seen generally, it is *noxious-stimuli* that bring the ground system (mesenchyme, RES, soft connective tissue) into a stress situation: injuries or mechanical disturbances, physico-chemical damage, poisons, and tissue-active hormones. Damage of this type comes via the skin (percutaneous, intracutaneous and subcutaneous), or is intramuscular; via the blood (in intravenous application); or intradural (CSF flooding *Speranski* 1950). The disturbance fields appear at these ports of entry (disturbance fields), but only manifest themselves as such when local defence has broken down, or in other words, if the disturbance field starts to "spread", i.e. a distant effect develops. The *distant effect* can be general or local.

The disturbance field, to which insufficient attention is often paid, is the *digestive tract*, whose upper surface is exposed to the alimentary environment. This surface has an organ typical epithelium; according to the usual definition, the intestinal wall in the mucosa and submucosa is *lymphoreticular or soft* cellular tissue, with capillaries and nerve endings, and is rich in extracellular or lymphatic fluid. Nerves and vessels have – cum grano salis – no direct functional contact with the epithelium. The entire ground system exists in the tunica propria and submucosa of the gastrointestinal tract in its most pure form. If one considers what the human being expects from his digestive tract, it is no wonder that the intestinal system is often the largest *disturbance area*, and – as I have seen in patients myself – that diseases (allergies, eczema, etc.) resist therapy until the disturbances and their general effects, the intestinal flora and function, are cured.

It was only possible to establish disturbances of the intestinal flora with precision after 1982. Only then did it become possible to investigate all four levels of the possible disturbances from the fresh, warm stool: cultures and quantity determination of aerobic and anaerobic microorganisms and fungi, as well as investigations for protozoa and nematods. These investigations were carried out by Prof. *J. Thurner* (in Vienna since 1982) and her co-workers, and we owe them our thanks.

Up to the middle of 1987, about 1.700 complete stool cultures had been carried out, and showed a totally varying picture in intestinal microorganism aberrations, with consequences for the total defense process. A differentiation has to be made between primary and secondary disturbances of the balance of the intestinal flora. The primary ones are predominant; the secondary ones are the consequence of extra-abdominal defense insufficiency, and are thus more difficult to treat.

Primary intestinal flora aberrations arise from a variety of causes, mainly as a consequence of gastric acid deficiency (no disinfection of uncooked food), as a late consequence of severe intestinal infections (e.g. after dysentery, typhus and food poisoning), after antibacterial therapy (antibiotics, sulfonamides, imidazole due to damage to normal intestinal symbiosis, and alteration of the intestinal milieu due to fungal infestation).

Secondary disturbances of the balance of the flora occur in severe disturbances of the total defence performance – in cancer patients, after immunosuppresive therapy, in the late stages of inflammatory diseases (e.g. in TB, and the end stages of PCP and MS), and in inherited and acquired immune deficiency. There are many types of intestinal flora disturbance. In 4.6% of the investigations there is a complete deficiency of Escheria coli and in 41.7% a complete deficiency of the lactic-acid-forming Lactobacillus acidophilus and Bacterium bifidum, or a serious reduction in the numbers of these normal intestinal symbiotics. Escheria coli produces, among other substances, *Pischinger's* monocyte factor, which is important for the activation of the function of *Peyer's* plaques and the intestinal lymph nodes (formation of lymphocyte factor). The lactic-acid-forming Lactobacillus acidophilus and Bacterium bifidum have two important physiological roles; previous experience shows that their deficiency leads to inhibition of absorption of minerals, particularly of trace elements (especially Fe and Zn), and they are necessary for the maintenance of normal intestinal flora relationships. Since we have been able to establish the quantity relationships of these symbiotics for about 1 year, it has been shown that not only total deficiency is important; a reduction in the lactic-acid-forming microorganisms is also important.

Apart from this deficiency of normal symbiotics, there is a palette of pathogenic microorganisms, and decomposition and fermentation microorganisms, in both the aerobic and anaerobic flora.

Obligate pathogens (pathogenic Coli strains, Pseudomonas aeruginosa; α and β hemolytic Streptocci and hemolytic and non-hemolytic Staphylococcus aureus) were present in 21% of all the stool cultures. Aerobic strains disturbing the balance of the flora were found in 80.1% of the cultures, and anaerobic strains with this effect in 76.8% of the cultures. At the same time, this means that mixed disturbances of the balance of the flora are uncommonly frequent, and that, mainly, only some of the microorganisms are affected. It has to be emphasized that the patients' subjective complaints are generally more severe with anaerobic disturbances of the normal flora than those with isolated aerobic disturbances. This is completely understandable, as the anaerobic share of the total intestinal flora is about 90%.

Fungi (mainly Candida albicans, but also Candida spec. and parapsilosis, Trichosporum spec., Geotrichum spec., Rhodotorula spec., and Torulopsis spec.) are found in 61.2% of all cultures. the pathogenic effect depends on the quantity present; quantities of 10^2 fungi/g stool are not clinically relevant; the first problems appear with quantities from less than 10^3 org/g stool.

Fungal quantities between below 10^3 and above 10^5 set off disturbances that are graded as toxic. In addition, the food decomposition products, the metabolic products of the fungi themselves, and the fermentation of carbohydrates, particularly sugar, are important. From more than 10^6 org/g, there are more and more inflammatory (colitic) symptoms. It is therefore important for the clinical diagnosis to determine both the quantity and quality of the fungal presence.

Among the protozoa, Lamblia infections were surprisingly common. Between 1983 and 1985 a massive wave of these infections spread over Europe – some of our own patients lived in the most northerly part of Schleswig Holstein – and not less than 32% of the cases had Lamblia cysts in the stool. The number of positive cases only fell to 13.2% after the rigorous winter of 1986/87. In contrast all the other protozoa (apathogenic Entamoeba coli, Isospora belli and Sarcocystis species) are found extremely seldom (in a total of 19 cultures), but from the metabolic point of view, they are as important as Lambliasis.

Worms and worm eggs are found increasingly seldom today. Oxiuriasis (in children) and ascariasis have only been found in 4% of the investigations.

However, all these disturbances in the balance of the intestinal flora – particularly the mixed forms – lead to important disturbances of defense performance capacity. This has three important consequences:

1. Resorption disturbances (vitamins, minerals, trace elements), whereby Lamblias are particularly important nutrition parasites,

2. Toxins (metabolic products of intestinal flora imbalance, decomposition strains, and fermentation substances),

3. Blockade of the abdominal lymph apparatus by toxins and living microorganisms.

The intestinal tract can thus become the most extensive disturbance field for the regulatory system, and stresses the ground system through toxins and mineral deficiencies, since this tissue is most abundant in the abdomen, and is present there in its purest form.

Primary disturbances of intestinal flora balance can be healed in a few weeks or months by specific therapy of the obligate pathogenic microorganisms, the large quantity of fungi and protozoonoses, and subsequent control of symbiosis with dextrorotatory lactic acid and freeze-dried intestinal symbiotics and some patience.

However, this is not the case with secondary disturbances. We understand these as being the defence disturbances of extraabdominal origin, whose primary causes have already been described. These disturbances lead to a spiral of negative effects, for the primary disturbance is intensified by the secondary disturbance of the balance of the flora. Healing is only brought about with simultaneous, successful immune stimulation.

Correction of the pH, the intestinal flora relationships and intestinal function is – as already introduced by *Pischinger* (1975) – important for the success of regulatory therapy. In chronic diseases the intestinal flora relationships are only normal in 2.5% of the patients; in 97.5% the imbalance is more or less severe. It should not be forgotten that gastric acid deficiency and ferment insufficiency, for example after diseases of the liver and pancreas, have to be treated at the same time in order to prevent a general recurrence of the imbalance of the flora.

The same applies to the chronic disturbance fields that are common in daily practice: the ENT, dental and faciomaxillary areas, chronic appendicitis, cholecystitis, and badly healed scars which can often cause "Huneke's secondary phenomenon" as well as the usual disturbance fields.

Like the entire science of disturbance fields, the "secondary phenomenon" cannot be understood until one has understood the total ground system with its three "assisting poles": the nerves (midbrain), the cell (lymphatic tissue) and the hormone pool (adrenals).

Understanding of the phenomenon came from 1. the development of serum *iodometry* and *electrometry* for examining the processes in the ground system, 2. the discovery of the puncture phenomenon as evidence of the total reaction of the ground system, 3. recognition that the ground system determines the reaction situation and the type of reaction, 4. that the ground system reacts quickly and that the main function of the system is directed at polarization and depolarization, and 5. that every disturbance field event take place primarily in cellular connective tissue, identical with the ground system, and that such processes lead to changes of tissue potential, which brings the complete nonspecific autonomic system into play. Thus, when a "spreading" disturbance field is present somewhere, the total ground system is disturbed, as our bilateral iodometry tests (with *Kellner*) show, although not to the same extent everywhere. First of all, general complaints appear. If an organ is affected by an additional specific noxious event that is so strong that it cannot be overcome, the relevant local damage appears, e.g. in the liver, pancreas, kidney, lung, gastrointestinal tract, etc., as well as joints, tendons and similar organs.

Eppinger (1949) discusses these processes: he sees the general disturbance as a disturbance of permeability, with albuminuria in the tissues.

If *Impletol, Kofficain, Xyloneural or Elpimed* are injected into a "guilty" depolarization center which are substances that repolarize, it can be understood that the total, general situation can return to normal. The defence capacity is restored as far as possible. Consequently, altered organ functions that are distant from the basic focus, as well as general and local symptoms, are thus restored to normal provided that – in general – the normalization in the disturbance field persits, or general regulation has been restored to the extent that the disturbance field influence – termed *false* spread – can be overcome.

According to the measurements made by Professor *Kracmar* (1961), under constant conditions in a column 9 mm in diameter and 15.4 mm long (in a Pravaz injection), Factor M (1.2%) has an R = 0.95 kilo-ohms and a C = 1.9 µF, Impletol (2%) R = 2.1 kilo-ohms and a C = 1.1 µF, and Xyloneural (1%) R = 1.4 kilo-ohms and C = 1.01 µF. All three substances have an ergometropic and polarizing effect.

From the same point of view, the effect of *a paravenous* injection can also be understood: the surroundings of the vessel, the perivascular tissue, with its abundant nerve content, which has been described for ages as soft connective tissue, is a classical autonomic ground system. With Impletol or Xyloneural infiltrations, a hyperpolarized imbalance here is made into a *depolarized field. There should be no difficulty in understanding the intravenous Impletol injection.* Obviously, even if it only lasts a short time, the resulting alteration of the milieu is sufficient to cause leukocyte reactions through leukolysis, and to alter the energy situation in the perivascular and interstitial tissue through capillary permeability, and thus also in the ground system.

Sometimes one comes across a version of *Huneke's* phenomenon where there is an *immediate* reciprocal effect between the disturbance field and the distant diseased site, and discusses the possibility of a specific distribution of Impletol to diseased areas from the treated disturbance field. I hope to have shown that the secondary phenomenon is a matter of a general retuning in the total biological ground system with the bioelectrical (oxydoreductive) potential as the central point, and all the consequences in blood and tissue. This must also lead to restitution in the diseased major reaction point – so far as this is anatomically possible. The patient finds the change in the situation at these points.

The secondary phenomenon was explained objectively to this extent by *Pischinger* in 1961, and taken into consideration by *Huneke*. In 1968, the objectivation (*Stacher* [1966]) was examined once more, and later a few times more (e.g. *Bergsmann* see contributions), with the effect and result that the secondary phenomenon could be explained more clearly of the structure of the autonomic field is considered – as I explain. From these papers, I would like to extract observations made by *Stacher* on the *side-effects* in the secondary phenomenon. This deals with bioelectrical measurements in scars. *Schoeler* (1960), *Kracmar* (1961) and *Stacher* (1966) had already demonstrated that scars have a false potential. *Stacher* carried out observations on appendix scars that were disturbance-free, and others that had a disturbance field effect. He writes the following about these scars: "with the help of a simple tube voltmeter, we measured the skin resistance between a ring-shaped electrode on the lower leg immediately under the knee and individual points on the scar and the surrounding skin." With a disturbance-free appendix scar "there was no great difference between the measuring point and the points on the surrounding skin." The values were between 100 and 150 kilo-ohms. "In contrast, at the measuring point, the scars with a disturbance field effect had a resistance of up to 1,400 kilo-ohms more than the surrounding skin; the surrounding skin measuring points were not more than 1 mm distant from the scar.

Stacher also points out: "Afterwards, we carried out random measurements on a series of scars that gave no clear clinical impression of being disturbance fields, and found such resistance differences more often than expected. This is parallel with the histological investigations that *Kellner* (1963, 1969) carried out independently on a wide variety of scars, since the histological criteria for a focus were present in a high percentage of the scars. These scars are therefore to be regarded as potential disturbance fields. In our resistance measurements, there was also the interesting fact that when the measurements were carried out several times in the same way, depending on atmospheric influences, they varied; in the scars the varations were much greater than in simultaneous hand-to-hand measurements. It can be assumed from this that the disturbed scars, and probably every other disturbance field, have a "battery" effect, in the pure physical sense.

Stacher gives some examples of coincidence between infiltration of a disturbance field with Impletol, etc. and the clinical reaction. However, he does not always find the breakdown of high resistance to be connected with the secondary phenomenon. A *late reaction* can also take place – 1 hour after the injection, according to Stacher. The term "secondary phenomenon" therefore has to be taken with a grain of salt. We should perhaps use the term *Huneke* phenomenon, thus providing both brothers with an appropriate memorial.

Stacher points out the correctness of the statement made by W. Huneke (1983) that it is often the case that only individual areas of the scar act as disturbance fields and that one should infiltrate the entire scar if measurents are not possible.

With these and other examples, *Stacher* confirms that the distant effects of an active disturbance field can be made to disappear when the bioelectrical conditions are normalized. It should not be overlooked that the secondary phenomenon is also the main evidence for the reality of the opposite process, namely the falsely-named "spread" effect, proceeding from altered areas of the ground system. The research results already discussed provide an explanation. This is a *total energy reaction* that leads to a general or local disturbance field effect, and its being broken off is based on the secondary or late phenomena.

To conclude this chapter, it can be pointed out that the substances that can be detected by serum iodometry (*Pischinger* 1975) allowed the basis of humoral regulation in the autonomic ground system to be recognized for the first time, assessed quantitatively, and generally explained according to chemistry and mechanism of action.

When the total biological ground system, its characteristics and effects have been recognized and taken into account, hardly any theoretical or practical medical problem will be met that cannot also be regarded from this basis.

To conclude this presentation, 5 brief examples should be given from which the role of the total biological ground system with the humoral factor (ELPIMED) is clarified in the organism and medicine. The first example affects cardiac crises, the second carcinoma, the third apoplexy, the fourth the manifestations of old age, and the fifth the problem of mild x-ray irradiation according to *R. Pape.*

Theory and clinical practice provide a long series of autonomically controlled functions. For our purposes, it is sufficient to emphasize the important points about regulation. It is, as the term "vital nerves" (L.R. Müller 1931) (*A. Bethe* 1952) brought out, the control of the unconscious vital functions. With these – according to the teachings of biology and general physiology – energy is in the foreground: physical and physico-colloid-chemical processes. The permeability relationships and bioelectrical potentials are connected with these.

The primary heart problems today are *myocardial infarction* and myocardial damage. As regards their cause, there are two opinions – as I said at the Heidelberg symposium: arteriosclerosis and the cardiac muscle theory. The latter see the cause of the infarct, even if complex, as not being in processes that narrow the arteries, but in primary damage to the myocardium of the left ventricle. *Kern* (1974), with older and newer authors (*Manfred v. Ardenne*) set damage of the muscle fibers at the beginning of the pathological process. Through further insult (stress and risk factors) that prevent restitution, or minimize it, the primary damage becomes worse, and finally leads the coronary arteries to disaster.

The key question is what prevents the healing and restitution of damaged cardiac muscle. The studies by *Buchner* and co-workers show that *hypoxia* in the myocardium leads to focal changes. *Kern* and the other defenders of the cardiac muscle theory also include an inhibition of oxygen utilization in the causes of disturbed restitution. *W.R. Hess* (1948), *H. Eppinger* (1949), *Sarre* (1953) and especially *K. Wetzler* show that oxygen utilization is a function of autonomic regulation. In parasympathetic tone it is increased; in sympathetic tone it is reduced. Disturbances of the latter type must favor cardiac muscle damage. It should also be considered that in the heart, as in other organs, there is no individual innervation via synapses. Here too, the control takes place through the entire ground system. If disturbances in this ubiquitous system affect the entire organism, then the heart cannot be excluded. The disturbance factors include general factors, e.g. excessive, long-lasting physical or psychic stress. However, the possibilities that occur in daily practice should not be excluded, which can also participate in the complex of infarction causes as local disturbance fields (*Rudich* [1972], *Pischinger* [1975]).

Similar considerations affect the cancer problem. In cancer patients, serum iodometry always shows regulatory inhibition. This is caused and maintained not only by "foci" or disturbance fields, e.g. in the head area, but also by other disturbed sites in the ground system, for example, originating in the *intestine*, whose entire mucosa shows the typical structure of a ground system. Naturally, in individual cases it cannot be shown whether disturbances are caused by the tumor, or were already present and favored the presence of pathological cells, or whether the defense has hindered the formation of "autochthonous" cancer cells. Here, a statement by F. *Perger* (1972) is interesting, where he reported that 25% of his patients with "regulatory paralysis" developed a tumor in later years. In any case, the participation of regulatory disturbances in the course of cancer cannot be ignored. The behaviour of the connective tissue in the tumor and around it leaves no doubt about this. The state of the normal parenchymal cells includes altered cancer cells and their energy (*Ruthenstrodt-Bauer* et al. [1966], *Seeger* [1943]).

Many individual questions remain open in this field. For example, whether and what connections exist between leukolysis as an autonomic function and cytolysis according to *Freund* and *Kaminer* (1925) and if this could be investigated.

Some important basic points emerge from the above as regards non-surgical cancer treatment, apart from early diagnosis and early operation: 1. Clearing of all disturbance foci so far as possible, 2. Restoration of regulatory and defense capacity through targeted after-treatment to activate the ground system in order to avoid stress and damage from the operation and massive irradiation, 3. Avoidance of general stress and damage caused by drugs.

In my opinion (*Pischinger* 1961), in concomitant cancer therapy, apart from the points mentioned above, a basic rule is that the *defense* capacity of the ground system has to be reinforced as much as possible in the direction of tissue respiration. This alone is connected with weakening the tumor cells. The prospect of successful direct tumor therapy is given only by contact irradiation, either with x-rays or radium, applied directly to the tumor. If this is not the case, more "healthy" tissue will be irradiated also, or affected by drugs, e.g. cytostatics, in such a way that one must always bear in mind that important defense tissues will be affected and damaged with every type of therapy.

A few more important points have to be made about radiotherapy. Many years ago F. *Perger* (1958) was able to show on a large group of patients that the size of a radiation effect large enough for lung screening, a film and orthogram, causes a reduction in serum calcium, a change which he recognized as being as significant as a shock effect in his regulation studies. Apart from this, there is a dissociation between the normally parallel courses of the calcium and cholesterol values. I then investigated *Pape's* weak radiation with the spectrographic 3-hour test on protein-free serum extract. A midbrain irradiation with 5 R skin dosage gives an increase of the UV-absorbing substances in the critical range after one hour. After 3 hours, they are practically back at the original level. After irradiating the sacral field with 150 R the spectrogram reacts differently. In the first hour after radiation, there are no changes in the spectrogram; a greater alteration appears after 3 hours. In the first case, the critical substances are released rapidly; in the second case they disappear. Whether by oxidation or another system has not been decided. The important point about this weak radiation is that the changes brought about in regulation are so minor that the organism can overcome them on its own. This treatment is thus like a mild push at the defense system, without producing blockade. One keeps hearing from medical practitioners who use this method that it is one of the best additional treatments in cancer (*Zabel* [1941] *Riccabona* [1954]; personal informants). Incidentally, midbrain-hypophysis short-wave-flooding according to *Schliephake* and *Samuels* (1952) belongs to this type of therapy; here, the emphasis of the therapy is on the midbrain.

Normal radiotherapy with high doses seems not to be without disadvantages, since it stresses the ground system to a significant extent. *Kellner* et al. 1971 have undertaken to follow-up the autonomic ground situation in cancer patients who have received long-term radiotherapy with the usual doses, with the help of serum iodometry *(Pischinger)* using the *Kellner* and *Klenkhart* (1970) method. There was a continuing reduction of the IUV in the methanol serum extract. The attempt to correct the loss of unsaturated fatty acids with injections of "Essential"® *(Nattermann)* strengthened the effect. On the other hand, it could be avoided by injecting 1 ml ELPIMED before each irradiation. This corresponded to the practical experience that the radiology "headache" can be prevented with ELPIMED. These types of treatment show that both the mild intervention in the midbrain and that in the periphery initiate a total reaction which is expressed in serum iodometry over the next few hours. With the midbrain, it is so minor that it can be corrected in a few hours. This *substance* in the autonomic ground system is the chemical expression of the good effect of the therapy. Naturally, favorable effects cannot be obtained at once. All these facts indicate how important it is not to ignore biological-medical treatment in tumors. One of these several treatments is *Leupold's* method, which is not only misunderstood, but actively disfavoured. I have known this treatment for a long time, and since reading *Leupold's* book, I can make sense of it. I found out that *Leupold's*

(1954) instructions were followed by a group of internal medicine specialists without success. In practice, I got to know the technique from the Hainburg physician, Dr. R. *Plohberger*; he has mastered the technique, and knows where others have made mistakes. Naturally, it is irrevelant to prove mathematically that not a single salt molecule reaches a cell, with a given number of cells in the body and the use of a saline solution as strongly diluted as that required by *Leupold* (1954). With *Plohberger* (1972), I saw what the *Leupold* therapy can do when it is carried out exactly according to instructions.

It is assumed that this therapy is known. Essentially, it consists of a preparatory period of 3 weeks with a carbohydrate-free diet. Then comes one day of glucose, starting with large quantities and then reducing, intravenously, three times a day. Finally, the carbohydrate is given as bread. Between the carbohydrate doses, the patient is given either insulin or *Leupold's* salt mixture. The treatment is called "alternating therapy" (Schaukeltherapie). *Leupold* uses the cholesterin to sugar and phospholipid test = Ch/Zp to evaluate the therapy.

Schaukeltherapie is not unknown. *F. Lutz* described one type: ELPIMED is given for two to three days subcutaneously; the next day there is a subcutaneous injection of 5–8 I.E. old insulin at the same time as white bread, to exclude a hypoglycemic effect; it is only a matter of the effect of the protein in the insulin. ELPIMED is ergotropic; the protein is tropotrophic. In most cases, regulatory paralysis can be interrupted with this treatment. The same effect is achieved by *Leupold's* game with sugar: insulin.

This method produces surprising results in other areas – not only in the treatment of tumors. Psoriasis is an indication. Even severe general cases can be healed completely (*Leupold* 1954, *Plohberger* 1971). More interesting – but not surprisingly – patients who still have foci or disturbance fields have more resistance than the non-stressed according to the *Leupold* and *F. Lutz* treatment methods.

There is a whole series of other cancer treatments. They are summarized and dealt with a book by *Zabel*. Two others should be emphasized: *Gerson's* diet and treatment, which is mainly aimed at the intestine and liver; and overheating therapy (*Schlenz, Lampert* (1962) *Ollendiek*). According to the bioelectrical measurements made by *Hauswirth* (1973), and *Kracmar* (1971), warmth produces ergotropic effects.

An analysis of foci and disturbance fields seems to be essential; but the normal rules have to be followed, to prevent a worsening of the tumor situation. The removal of the "cancer load" is essential, but it puts the organism in danger, as. *H. M. Plohberger* (1972) has shown.

Whatever happens, the intestinal function has to be restored to normal, as the work by *Rusch* (1977, 1978) has shown; or other measures to restore the intestinal balance (*Gerlach* 1970, *Gerson* 1958) are undertaken.

Recently, the work done by *Wolff* has come into discussion. This deals with a fermentation product called WOBE MUGOS with high, but subtoxic concentrations of vitamin A.

ELPIMED is a great help in the treatment of cancer. I *(Pischinger)* have personally treated a patient with lung metastases after breast cancer and kept her relative free of discomfort for 2 years, until the terminal stages. Morphine had to be given in addition during the final few days. Other doctors have also reported on such cases *(H. Sommer)*. I also have case histories from Dr. *Karl Singer* of Bad Vöslau; after consultations with Dr. *Lutz* and myself both his operable and inoperable patients are given 1 ccm ELPIMED and 500 γ Vitamin B 12 every two days; post-menopausal patients may also be given a daily C. luteum tablet (Orgamatril). *Singer* reports on 40 patients: 13 have died up to now, including 8 with survival times of between 8 and 21 years. Naturally the major disturbance areas were removed and dietary control was used.

Fresh cell therapy and hematogenous oxidation were also used. I got to know both methods personally. In experiments with guinea pigs I saw that the injected tissue material became necrotic and was broken down. In the end, a connective tissue scar remains. It has been reported that the adrenal hormones increase after cell injection. To me, this seems to be a sign of increased stress *(Selye)*.

I was able to study hematogenous oxidation more precisely with *H. Wehrli*. I *(Pischinger)* found the following: with hematogenous oxidation according to *F. Wherli*, the oxygen loading of the erythrocytes seems to have less significance in the effects than the simultaneous irradiation with UV light and its influence on the leukocytes. The venous blood is loaded with oxygen in the equipment, a process that also takes place in the lungs. Fully oxygenated blood flows in the arteries, provided severe lung or blood damage is not present. It is therefore difficult to see the purpose of loading venous blood with oxygen. If the change in the leukocyte content after flooding with oxygen and UV irradiation is followed, which resembles ozone treatment – as one recognizes from the smell – there are major differences between the cell count from the blood taken from the vessel before the treatment and the blood after the application of oxygen and UV light. The following table gives information on this. It concerns blood from patients with a variety of chronic diseases. Two samples were of conserved blood (K). The numbers before the oblique stroke are from untreated blood, and the numbers following from blood after oxygenation and UV:

1. 5622/3749
2. 4052/4155(K)
3. 7859/7055
4. 5317/3997
5. 6067/4962
6. 5988/6155
7. 5483/5071(K)
8. 5903/5551
9. 4204/3447
10. 1723/1601
11. 6038/5255
12. 6967/6551
13. 9545/8763
14. 4388/4574
15. 6502/4585

The blood is reinfused after the treatment.

The difference between the two mean values (the values before and after the oblique) is minus 999.4. The t-difference test shows a probability of error between the two states (mean values) of less than $P = 0.001$, so there is high significance.

The question is what causes this major loss of leukocytes; this is also described by *Storck* (1954) in his studies on rheumatism as a regulatory disease with other marked appearances. First, it has to be remembered that leukocytes remain stuck on the glass walls. However this should not be over-evaluated, as the following observation shows. Trial by Dr. *U*: before, 4388; after oxygen ventilation alone 4547. So the leukocyte count remains the same. Only the combination of oxygen treatment with UV reduces the figure to 3557.

So we are left with only one reason for the fall in the cell count; forced leukolysis, as seen in the lysis forms before and after oxygenation with UV; before, 10% and 14% after oxygen plus UV.

The spectrogram of the protein-free serum extract changes also. However, this point has not been fully researched, only to the point that the fact has been established.

The well-regarded *Havelick*'s principle obviously also works according to the same principle; here, blood from the vein is irradiated with UV light in an open bowl, and shaken lightly (see in *Sehrt* 1942); then it is injected intravenously. The favorable effect is absent when there is no UV irradiation, or defibrinated blood or serum is irradiated and injected. These are facts that also indicate a reciprocal effect – leukocytes and UV irradiation.

In summary, hematogenous oxidation and analogous methods indicate that the favorable effects come from regeneration and activation of the blood by the lymphocytes (leukolysis) and the protein-free fraction of the serum, and not from loading the erythrocytes with oxygen. Once again, leukolysis is seen to be an important process for the regeneration of the organism.

Therapeutic Consequences of Ground Regulation Research

The consequences from the measurability of the ground function processes are extensive; but they are evolutionary and not revolutionary. It may be the case that everything in today's medicine could be turned upside down, as many traditionalists fear.

The course of a disease – as every previous generation of physicians knew – depends on the existing defense situation as well as the type and intensity of the noxious factors. The only new point is that the defense situation does not depend directly on the immune system, but on the ground system. However, it has to be pointed out that other regulatory systems are also involved in the defense processes, such as the autonomic nervous system and the hormone system, and that the distribution of tasks in the defense system should not be a surprise. Knowledge of the ground system and the fact that it can be measured do not replace specific diagnostic methods, but expand them in the sense of also paying attention to the irreplacable host defense performance. This is a special chance of therapy when the last noxious factors responsible are unknown or have not been demonstrated clearly. In particular, knowledge of the ground system can clarify the origins of multifactorial diseases more exactly than before. This opens up research into dimensions that have been unknown up to now. It has to be pointed out that those active in ground system research are also aware that everything has not yet been clarified, in spite of considerable progress.

In 1949, *Eppinger* had already given the opinion that disease begins in the extracellular matrix, and that an attack on the parenchymal cells is secondary. Specific symptoms – and thus specific diagnosis – only become possible with cellular change, at a relatively late stage when one considers the relatively long prodromal stages of many infections. However, determination of the defense situation, even in healthy subjects, can give advance indication of how an incipient infection will be combated and regulated.

To do this with an entire population is pure utopia, as everything would collapse for reasons of cost and personnel. But previous research has given important results on which factors have to be eliminated as much as possible to produce a general improvement in the health of the population. The close realtionship between ground and immune function, and the dependence of specific immune performance on the course of nonspecific regulation, give the possibility of retuning the immune system by rehabilitation of the ground system, or at least to get close to this. Delay in the otherwise normal course of immune reactions makes it possible, for example, for invasive microorganisms to adjust themselves to the milieu of the body and bring about chronic inflammation.

The aim of regulatory medicine is to restore normal defense function after treating the specific disease symptoms (acute infections, inflammatory systemic disease and after tumor load removal, etc.), to produce a positive influence on the further course of the disease. Only in this way can the patient be brought back to a state where recurrences, new outbreaks or metastases can be controlled. Rehabilitation of the regulatory system is – as already said – the only chance for normal healing, or at least improvement of the course, in diseases where the specific noxious factors are not known, or cannot be combated at the moment.

However, this rehabilitation of the defense regulatory system demands a certain change of thought in therapy, which can now take the regulatory system into account.

Selection of Specific Drugs and Avoidance of Delayed Effects

The selection of a specific therapeutic method only takes place according to the basic rule of the smallest stress to the ground functions – this corresponds to medical school teaching that methods with the least possible side-effects should be used. Mostly, side effects are due to a severe humoral shock reaction, which favors allergic reactions in particular. The use of a drug not only causes the shock reactions of the exogenous stimulus, but this affects the existing defense situation. Thus if there is a chronic state of humoral shock, it is strengthened by the exogenous substance. The importance of the ground system, which is initially very hard to understand for a physician with a specific way of thinking, is that it reacts nonspecifically and uniformly to all stimuli, and that stimuli of this type therefore have a summation effect. It is also incapable to differentiate between friend and foe (*Heine* 1987) – particularly not its cells, the fibroblasts.

Based on this knowledge, therapy can be controlled in such a way that the side-effects and later undesired effects of substances with a highly specific effect can be reduced.

The first example is treatment with phenylbutazone, which was the leading antirheumatic 20–30 years ago. Apart from its antiinflammatory and antirheumatic effects, it often had allergic and hemotological side effects, and was therefore controversial. Addition of the monocyte factor (ELPIMED®) to the phenylbutazone injection (IRGAPYRIN® or BUTAZOLIDIN®) produced both a subjectively strong reduction in pain and disappearance of the allergic reactions – we experienced no further complications, including no hematological disturbances. We select analgesics and antirheumatics for oral use on the basis that they affect the ground functions as little as possible, or not at all. Of these, the salicylates belong to the substances with the least effect on regulation – but they are not always succesful in achieving the desired specific results. In testing the ground system under the influence of drugs, Ibuprofen and indomethacin only show mild stress to ground regulation, and these substances are therefore generally safe for the treatment of the active stages of rheumatic diseases.

However, in spite of their intensive shock effect on the ground system, the corticoids cannot always be avoided, although corticoid therapy can be carried out with significantly less effect on the ground system and other regulatory systems (bone metabolism, insulin production, etc.) if the entire daily dose is given between six and eight o'clock in the morning. The natural cortisol level is at its highest at this time, and this improves drug tolerance significantly. We thank observation of the circadian rhythm to avoid side effects not only to ground system research, but also to classical academic physicians like *Bethge* (1971) and *Wittenberg* et al. (1973).

Immunosuppression with acothiaprine and cyclosporin, or aureotherapy is really paralysing for the ground system, and activation is hardly ever possible, even to a limited extent. It is only justified where rehabilitation of the regulatory system is no longer possible; from our point of view it is a resignative type of therapy when already used from the time of the first defense derailment that might be rehabilitated. It is certainly acceptable as the final step – rather in the sense of a palliative operation for cancer.

Antibiotics are another example of paying attention to side effects on the ground system. They are also an example of how delayed effects can be avoided with simple methods.

One often experiences the antibiotics that are effective in vitro are not effective in vivo. Once again, the cause was found tobe in the humoral shock phases or blockade of the ground system. Giving monocyte factor simultaneously prevents the reactions and leads to a full antibiotic effect; it also prevents allergic reactions, at the same time. This solves one of the two problems in antibiotic therapy.

The second problem, which often gives the patients severe problems, is the disturbance of the balance of the intestinal flora with the development of bacterial imbalances in the flora, and, particularly, intestinal mycoses. Since antibiotics – like the cells of the ground system – also cannot distinguish between friend and foe, the normal intestinal microorganisms are often damaged at the same time as the pathogenic strains. Since they are obtained from fungal extracts or from technical processes with similar properties, the intestinal lumen is fungus-prone. Bacterial and mycotic aberrations of the intestinal flora also lead to significant resorption disturbances for vitamins, trace elements and minerals in those affected. The resulting deficiency states lead to a further disturbance of the defense cycles: mineral deficiency has a direct effect on the ground substance transmitter function, since the molecular sieve of the proteoglycans is influenced directly (*Heine* and *Schaeg* 1979); trace element deficiency inhibits the enzymes of the neurotransmitters and specific antibody and immunoglobulin production.

Disturbances of the gut flora are an important stress factor for defence functions (*Perger* 1985), and are easy to avoid; simple after-treatment with dextrorotatory lactic acid and the addition of important intestinal flora symbiotics (E. coli, B. acidophilus, B. bifidum) prevents the development of these intestinal problems.

The fixed humoral shock reaction in recurrent systemic inflammation (e.g. inflammatory joint rheumatism, multiple sclerosis, ulcerative colitis, etc.) leads all too easily to reactions of an allergic type in both uninfluenced disease forms and against drugs. Antiallergic therapy with calcium and antihistamines is therefore indicated in the active stages of these diseases: with this, remissions can often be accelerated, and side effects from the necessary specific therapy forms prevented. As regards abundant use of calcium in exacerbations of MS, the objection is made that calcium lengthens the stimulating pathway and is therefore undesirable. On the other hand, the reduction in inflammatory edema and prevention of tissue destruction should be seen as more important.

In patients with inflammatory systemic diseases one keeps on seeing that even banal viral infections are able to damage the defense capacity to the extent that regulation against the main disease breaks down and new exacerbations appear. Therapy with human gamma-globulin, a generally recognized method, this danger can be prevented to a large extent: knowledge of the intensivation of the ground system disturbance and the delayed immune reaction it causes is very close to substitution of this type.

Some important examples suffice to make the possibilities for careful treatment of the disturbed defense functions understandable. Paying attention to the fact that even the most highly efficacious specific therapeutic agent initiates a humoral shock effect that can damage an already damaged regulatory cycle, and that it can intensify this damage even further, leads to a significantly lower rate of these reactions, whether they take the form of an allergic reaction or have an unfavorable effect on the further course of the disease.

Here, it must be pointed out that the preparatory trials before the introduction of a new therapeutic substance are carried out on healthy animals, and that such nonspecific side effects cannot be recorded as an intensification of defense disturbance for this reason. In spite of their outstanding effects on an exacerbation of inflammation, the disadvantage of many chemotherapeutic substances is that they can initiate a change from the type of course that can be rehabilitated to one of the chronic-progressive forms that can scarcely be influenced. For this reason, to avoid these events, strict control of the indications is needed for all these substances, whether they are true immunosuppressives or only work in the same direction.

Rehabilitation of Defense Capacity

Restoration of at least near normal defense functions is – as is shown by the 40 years of ground system research – the most important precondition for avoiding relapses. This can be seen in patients with MS, who can be treated successfully: two patients lived for 25 years and 30 years respectively without an exacerbation. After 25 years, one patient developed severe toxoplasmosis which was followed by an exacerbation; the second patient had a severe psychic shock after 30 years, which set off an exacerbation. This means that the causative noxious agents (slow viruses?) had been present in the body the entire time, but that the defense capacity had been raised to such a level that they only made themselves manifest again under extreme conditions. *Issels* astonishing successes in the treatment of hopeless cancer patients, which the author was able to check on site with the chairman of the Vienna Health Council, are evidence that rehabilitation of the defense functions has to be given the same value as specific therapy.

However, appropriate preconditions have to be created, for it is not possible to rehabilitate these functions in such a way that such an effect is achieved without prior removal of chronic stresses. Usually, these stresses do not have a direct causal relationship with the later main disease; they only prepare the milieu where they can become established. They are therefore *predisposing factors*, as *Urbach* (1935) had already formulated in connection with a variety of allergens.

According to the current state of knowledge, these are silent inflammations (regarded earlier as "foci" with a direct causal connection with the main disease), intestinal disturbances (all forms of symbiosis disturbance), subsymptomatic toxicoses and deficiency states. In addition there are the abacterial disturbance fields, and scars with disturbed wound healing, often with foreign body inclusions.

Once again, as with chemotherapy, attention is paid to the disturbed defense function and its low capacity to accept stress. Operations, e.g. tonsillectomy and extensive dental clearance and reconstruction procedures are therefore delayed until the capacity of the regulatory cycle to accept stress has been raised by correcting stresses that can be treated conservatively. This avoids the complications and operative incidents that brought the old focal research into bad reputation. After treating the acute stages of inflammatory systemic diseases, the next step is to deal with the stresses that can be removed by conservative methods; only then are the necessary operative measures carried out (*Perger* 1987).

Conservative Therapy to Relieve Stress on the Regulatory Cycles

In the presence of deficiencies of vitamins, trace elements and minerals, and where there are toxic stresses, operative procedures for silent, chronic inflammations often lead to disturbances of the healing process, and thus to the formation of residual "foci", jaw ostitis, scar abscesses in the tonsillar area, etc., and this is so common that the effect of such unprepared procedures seems to be at best extremely questionable. The procedure is carried out to make rehabilitation of the defense capacity possible, not simply because one wants to carry it out. The preconditions for a normal healing process therefore have to be created in advance.

The consequences of these stresses are so intermeshed that a separate description is practically impossible: they are the consequences of resorption disturbances through upset intestinal symbiosis and ferment insufficiencies, subsymptomatic toxicoses through disturbances of the detoxification functions, and vitamin, trace element and mineral deficiency states.

Deficiency states can be traced back to two causes: to inadequate quantities in food, and resorption disturbances in the digestive tract. Subsymptomatic toxicoses are mainly caused by environmental pollution and a disturbed detoxification function, which also depends on trace element deficiency.

Reduced availability in food is mainly due to the false nutrition of many people. However, with the example of zinc deficiency, one can see that even with the best intent in the world ideal nutrition may not be possible: *Seeling* et al. (1977) described the frequent appearance of zinc deficiency in calves that corresponded to human acrodermatitis enteropathica and also concerns extreme zinc deficiency. *Kostolics* (1979, personal information) reported on skin diseases in pigs in mass breeding units that could also be traced back to zinc deficiency. Since zinc is best resorbed from meat foods, there is no guarantee of an adequate supply under such conditions. If we limit ourselves to zinc, the consequences are considerble: in zinc deficiency, protein synthesis is inhibited, including DNA and RNA synthesis and immunoglobulin formation; zinc is absolutely essential for the activation of the polymerases. The detoxification function is also disturbed: the metalothionine responsible for the chelation and removal of toxic heavy metals cannot become sufficiently active, and with high-grade zinc deficiency there is almost always a reducation of the β-globulins and thus a considerable inhibition of detoxification processes.

In addition, zinc is functionally necessary for at least 80 enzymes, including the enzymes for the neurotransmitters and insulinase.

It can thus be seen clearly that a zinc deficit has considerable negative significance for healing processes – even if the immune system is more affected than the ground system in these cases, it still has the same significance for the rehabilitation of defense functions as the mineral deficiencies that affect the ground system directly.

In our experience, calcium deficiency is the most important mineral deficiency, followed by magnesium deficiency. These have a direct effect on the ground functions, but are very important for other regulatory cycles.

The function of the molecular sieve for transmitter function, described by *Heine* and *Schaeg* (1979) depends on the size of the pores, and its permeability for minerals of the extracellular matrix; it alters this to a great extent by taking-up or giving-off water, which is made possible by exchange of Na and K to Ca and Mg. With the many biological tasks of these minerals, even minor deficits are also important. In addition, minerals participate in the release of start-energy for the defense functions. Energy is obtained from the adenosine triphosphate acids by activation of AT-phosphates. All previous experience shows that these AT-phosphatases are inhibited by Mg and activated by Ca, so that energy release in the humoral shock phase is inhibited with raised Mg in the ground tissues and activated with the increase in Ca in the countershock phase. Here, the presentation by *Heine* was followed, so far as the localization of obtaining energy is concerned. The various activity grades of AT-phosphatases were taken from the reactive behaviour of the minerals in the various phases of the alarm reaction, which come from our own observations.

However, resorption disturbances in imbalances of symbiosis and dysfunctions in the digestive tract have greater significance for deficiency states than a reduced availability in nutrition. Even a deficiency of gastric acid leads to severe imbalances of symbiosis – no exception has been found up to now. Gastric acid is responsible for both the digestion of protein and disinfection of uncooked food, and this is responsible for the greater susceptibility to intestinal infection in states of subacidity or anacidity. This was also confirmed in susceptibility to Lambliasis of the intestine. Of 444 patients with this protozoal disease, none had hyperacidity; only 51 patients (11.5%) had normal acidity, and 393 (88.5%) had subacidity or anacidity (*Perger* 1988).

These examples show the importance of normal gastric acidity. Further experience on stool cultures of 1,700 patients showed that correction of intestinal relationships is not possible without HCl substitution – there is always a changing picture of bacterial and mycotic disturbances of symbiosis; the existing non-symbiotic strains have scarcely been eliminated when others establish themselves in the intestine.

There is however a point of view that HCl deficiency does not have to be corrected, as the pancreatic juices could break down the food protein without chylation by the gastric juices – but this doesn't appear to be completely true, due to the short time the food spends in the duodenum and the decaying processes in symbiotic disturbances. The disinfection function of gastric acid seems to have been overlooked in such opinions.

Resorption disturbances affect vitamins, trace elements and minerals. The demands made by the microorganisms in disturbed symbiosis for these substances for their own survival, particularly fungi and protozoa, reduce the amounts available for the host organism. This then leads to the secondary disturbances of defense and detoxification processes already described.

Incapacity for adequate detoxification and elimination has been investigated in detail (*Perger* and *Maruna* 1986, 1987, *Perger* 1987), in connection with the toxic heavy metals Pb, Cd and Hg, and partly with Ni. The conclusion was that inhibition of metalothionine in zinc deficiency scarcely leads to a picture of chronic poisoning, but that an interesting picture of enzyme disturbances can appear in the organism due to depot formation. *Maruna* and *Stipinovic* gave the first undeniable evidence in 1974 when they showed the cause of bone necroses after fractures to be an 8.2-times higher Pb content in the necroses as compared to normally-healing fractures. The formation of depots of Pb and Cd in bone leads to disturbances of its metabolism and can lead to severe consequences in a secondary injury, such as a fracture. Paradontosis with loosening of the teeth can also often be traced back to Cd depots in the jaw (*Perger* 1989). These problems are additional to the already-known damage to renal function (Cd) and intestinal colic (Pb).

In subsymptomatic intoxication elimination does not have to be as rapid as in marked intoxication, and chelation has important side effects (including loss of essential trace elements); two flies can be killed at the same time with zinc substitution: the deficiency state is normalized as regards other functions also, and activation of metalothionine leads to elimination of the toxic heavy metal, admittedly slowly, but carefully.

Vitamin deficiency can be demonstrated by a test injection. It is remarkable how activated the patients feel after such an injection. It consists of a combination of a water-soluble form of vitamin A, vitamin B complex and vitamin C (*Pancebrin Lilly*®). With persistent disturbances of intestinal symbiosis it is better to give the vitamin combination by injection in order to avoid giving the microorganisms causing the symbiosis disturbance an optimal supply also; later, the combination can be given orally. The initially astonishing activation effect of a vitamin injection gradually disappears, and disappears completely when the body depots are filled.

Deficiencies of Ca, Mg or Fe are replaced by oral medication.

Simple forms of intestinal symbiosis disturbance are solved primarily with dextrorotatory lactic acid and freeze-dried intestinal symbiotics. The consumption of bacterial preparations one and a half to two hours before the next meal is, however, recommended, to make their revitalization and adherence to the intestinal mucosa possible. The usual system immediately before the meal is often without success as the the food bolus carries the microorganisms with it, and they are excreted with the stool.

High-grade mycoses and protozoonoses are initially minimized by specific medication (antimycotics or imidazole derivatives), and this is followed immediately by the symbiosis guidance described. It is important to accept that antimycotics kill the fungi present, but do not alter the susceptibility of the intestine to fungi, and that imidazole eliminates both protozoa and anaerobic symbiotics – the milieu therapy that follows is therefore essential.

These measures for correcting deficiency states, the elimination of toxins, and normalization of the intestinal flora, produce an important relief of the stress on the nonspecific and specific regulatory systems, and improves their function towards the direction of normal function.

Elimination of Scar Disturbance Fields

The scar disturbance fields are still a controversial stress factor, as is their elimination with local anesthetics; neural therapy. Not every scar is a disturbance field with "distant effects". *Kellner* (1976) described the scars with a disturbance field effect as scars with disturbed wound healing, and confirmed this with impressive histological illustrations in operation scars with talcum crystal inclusions. In our own field we also found other inclusions, such as missile splinters and cloth remnants in war wounds; in accident scars there were often grains of sand, glass splinters and pieces of asphalt, etc. These inclusions can only be broken down slowly, or not at all. However they cause acidosis of the surrounding tissue and thus a change in ground regulation. Like silent, chronic inflammation, they can cause distant effects, and here there is an astonishing relationship with the acupuncture meridians, which affects the localization of the distant effects.

Infiltration of such scars with local anesthetics (procaine or lidocaine) is followed by repolarization of cell membranes, and this is maintained far beyond the local anesthetic effect. Through this, as *Kellner* (1976) described, blockage of the ground system is broken down. In this way, the disturbance can be broken down or at least regulated out. Repolarization of the cell membranes is a pure biological effect, but it is important for initiating all succeeding biological functions, including those of a biochemical nature.

The local anesthetic effect of procaine and lidocaine is essential for this effect. However, it should be regarded as an *additional* positive factor, since it leads to a pain-free reactivation of the defense functions. This exclusion of the distant effect of abacterial disturbance fields is also able to improve the defense state.

Relief of Silent Chronic Inflammation (Foci)

Only when the deficiency states have been corrected, the intestinal flora relationships at least generally normalized, the toxins eliminated and the scar disturbance fields eliminated, is operative elimination of the silent bacterial progresses free of risk, with a guarantee of no inhibition or disturbance of the healing processes.

The important effect of the so-called foci is not caused by the microorganism content. The spread of bacteria and toxins has a minimal role in their effect – this spread only plays a role in about 3.3% of cases, initiating septic or allergic reactions; in 96.7% the real mechanism resembles that of the abacterial disturbance fields. In addition, the constant demands on energy and substance to limit and localize the infection have to be taken into account; they are needed to hinder septic spread. This was shown on 7148 patients (*Perger* 1978, 1983). Existing silent, chronic inflammations therefore do not have to be eliminated because of their spread, but because of their energy-consuming limitation and tissue acidosis with increased fibroblast consumption.

Despite previous improvement of the defense state by the measures described above, the way patients with foci react is still so disturbed that the timing of the individual procedures has to be arranged in such a way that no overloading can occur due to a rapid series of operative shocks. In the heyday of focal therapy (about 1910 to 1940), elimination was carried out as rapidly and radically as possible, under the assumption of a direct-causal relationship between the focus and the secondary disease. However, this false point of view in the focal theory of that time (focal infection or focal allergy and focal toxicosis) often led to significant complications and long-term damage. The overloading of the already severely damaged ground system due to summation of operation shock often led to a final blockade of ground regulation and a change to chronic-progressive courses, and also to fatal incidents (particularly in septic forms), because the damaged defense circuit was no longer able to respond adequately to these stresses.

The timing of the necessary operations therefore has to made in such a way that the organism has enough time for recovery between the individual procedures. At the same time, a protective therapy is needed that checks the allergic-type overreaction, but does not suppress the healing processes.

Aiginger and *Neumayer* (1950) relate this recovery time to the possible appearance of serum sickness. This can appear until up to 21 days after a foreign protein injection – mostly, an organism needs just as long to recover from an operation or accident shock. This parallel between two basically completely different stresses shows the uniformity of the ground functions regarding all stimuli, and their significance as starters of normal or pathological defence processes. Incidentally, the existence and functions of the ground system were not known to the two authors at that time.

This means that the intervals between individual operative procedures have to be at least 4 to 5 weeks, to avoid overload reactions.

The task of protective therapy is to prevent an allergy-type reaction. It is therefore carried out with antiallergic substances; with calcium and antihistamines. This does not inhibit the normal healing processes.

The use of corticoids for protective therapy would be controversial as suppression of the healing processes would promote the formation of residual foci (tonsillar scar abscesses, jaw ostitis, etc.). With regard to antibiotics as protective therapy, *Riccabona* (1958) has already pointed out that this favors allergic reactions and the desired simultaneous immune stimulation is suppresed.

The aim of elimination of silent chronic inflammation is relief for the sick organism. Simultaneous activation of the defense and healing processes is an additional effect which is important and should not be suppressed. Only the allergy-type overreaction should be checked.

Rehabilitating After-treatment

The sick organism is not freed from its stresses by the measures described up to now; with the exception of a few early cases, the recovery of the regulatory system needs a long time; too long, under todays living conditions, to avoid the danger of new stresses and foci building up. Our own observations show that spontaneous rehabilitation needs two to three years.

Up to then there is a response to every infection and stimulus in the existing regulatory derailment, although to a lesser extent; the formation of new foci and development of chronic inflammation can't be avoided – with this the spiral of a complicated disease begins again, up to a fresh development of activation of the inflammatory systemic disease. It is therefore necessary to rehabilitate the defence functions in order to bring the reaction capacity of the regulatory system back to as normal a state as possible.

It would be too much to describe all the possible forms of therapy, but they all work most intensively on the ground system, and partly on the other systems (immune, autonomic and hormone systems).

Balneology and acupuncture have stood the test for over 2,000 years, although their effects on ground regulation were not known. Homeopathy in the hands of an expert has also stood the test for over 200 years, and its effects can be described as "informative". In addition there is neural therapy for restoration of the normal interface potentials and stimulation therapy (nonspecific stimuli, fever therapy, ozone therapy, etc.) and semispecific desensitization with foreign vaccines or autovaccines. In experienced hands they are all capable of restoring the defense functions to normal and can raise the stimulation threshold for totality reactions to the peripheral regulatory capacity in normal people of 500,000 microorganisms per vaccine or a corresponding stimulus equivalent. This stimulus threshold was tested on a wide variety of diseases, with 917 tests – only the healthy subject reacts initially to a stimulus of this level with a brief general reaction; all the chronically ill react with a 1/10 to 1/1000 with their already deranged totality reaction.

The choice of rehabiltation therapy can be left to the judgement and competence of the doctor carrying out the treatment. In nonspecific response of the ground system to stimuli the choice of therapy should be according to personal knowledge and experience rather than unnecessary special method.

Success and Failure in Regulatory Therapy

Particularly in inflammatory systemic diseases whose last initiating noxious agent is not clearly known and a specific therapy is not possible, restoration of normal defense functions is currently the only chance for healing or defect healing. It is important that a capacity for rehabilitation still exists, and with our current possibilities this is not always the case.

Immediate allergies, which cannot be controlled by currently used desensitization with the specific allergen are particularly suitable for treatment, also from the aspect of a disturbed defense situation. In many of our patients the appropriate investigations gave a series of predisposing factors such as chronic silent inflammation, deficiency states, and even heavy metal loading (particularly common with Hg, without this necessarily being a specific allergen). 220 patients out of 260 with allergies could be kept free of attacks with rehabilitation therapy (*Perger* 1978), namely 84.6%.

In exacerbation forms of inflammatory systemic disease (inflammatory rheumatism, MS, ulcerative colitis etc.) no further exacerbations were observed in 82% of the patients over an observation period of 8–30 years. Out of 1,136 patients with seronegative obligoarthritis and polyarthritis, only 204 patients had relapses, mainly due to the development of new foci or severe acute disease; but only 19 of the patients in this group could no longer be influenced by regulation. Up to now, 121 patients with multiple sclerosis have been treated, and apart from 22, all remained free of exacerbations in the observations period. The picture with chronic-progressive diseases is completely different and much less favorable; due to increased risk with operative procedures, many of these patients cannot be helped with this therapy, and with those where the possibility existed, rehabilitation of defense was only achieved in 18%; in 82% it was not achieved – apart from this, we are dealing here with defect healing, since irreversible tissue changes cannot be reversed with this treatment.

However, it can be seen from the almost 40 years of ground regulation research that a genuine healing of chronic diseases leading to restoration of the normal harmonious functions of the defense circuits is possible. All experience shows that without normalization of the ground regulation as starter of the defense processes, this cannot be attained. Mainly, the cellular and humoral immune reactions are not so strongly disturbed that they cannot take their normal course after normalization of the ground functions. The pituitary-adrenal axis recovers, as do the vascular nervous functions when attention is paid to the cybernetic aspect of the ground function and it is rehabilitated. At present, there is no possibility of restoring these regulations only where the ground system is irreparably blocked – particularly in chronic, progressive processes.

It must be added that blocking of the ground system can be overcome in some patients with malignant tumors, but the failure rate is higher than in PCP, and the number of cases is too small to awake hope; malignancies involve failure of the entire defense system – paralysis of the ground functions, and particularly, failure of the cellular immune reactions.

It is nothing new that healing of chronic disease is only possible through normalization of the defense functions: the old rule that a chronic inflammation only heals via an acute stage is, as before, topical. The basic rules on how this can be be done without serious risk, and in serious diseases such as systemic inflammation and malignancies, have been laid by *Pischinger*. His successors and students are charged with the tasks of solving the problems that remain open, and to bring the problems of defense upsets so far in the foreground as they can. The intermeshing of the regulatory system (biocybernetics) only works normally when the start takes place in the intercellular substance with adequate, energy-rich intensity and speed. To avoid misunderstandings, it has to be emphasized that humoral diagnosis and therapy should not replace the specific – but it presents the chance of expanding therapy beyond the specific, and should be given the same priority.

There is an important conclusion from these investigations. The first reaction at the site of the noxious agent invasion is marked by both biochemical (humoral) reactions and a change in the Ph to acidosis.

This biophysical reaction is the same for all exogenous stimuli, not only living agents. Bacteria, protozoa, viruses, toxins, trauma and ionising radiation can all produce the same effect. The important nonspecific reaction of initiating humoral shock can lead to exhaustion of ground regulation from the summation of all the stimuli, and be responsible for the pathological facts of other exogenous stimuli. This knowledge offers us the first concrete chance of getting to the bottom of multipathological processes – and that is the most important clinical aspect of *Pischinger*'s ground regulation research.

Literature

Achard, Ch. und *Feuillie, E.*: Sur la resistance leukozytaire. C. R. Soz. Biol. 59, 795 (1907).
Adler, E.: Erkrankungen durch Störfelder im Trigeminusbereich. 3., verb. Aufl. Verl. f. Medizin Dr. Ewald Fischer, Heidelberg 1983.
Aiginger, J., Neimayer E.: Die Beziehungen der Multiplen Sklerose zu anderen medizinischen Disziplinen. Klin. Med. (1951) 2.

Aschoff, L.: Pathologische Anatomie. 3. Aufl., Jena 1913.
–, – und *Kiyono:* Ein Beitrag zur Lehre von den Makrophagen. Verh. d. dtsch. Path. Ges. 16, 107 (1913).
Auböck, L.: Innervationstypen in der menschlichen Appendix. Acta histochemica Suppl. X, 225–231 (1967).
Baroldi, G.: Histopathological study of the intramural artery vessels in relation to the pathology of extramural coronary arteries myocardial damage. Cardiologia 41, 364–380 (1962).
Bennel, N. V. C.: Physiology of electronic junction. Ann. N. Y. Acad. Sci. 37. 509–539 (1966).
Bergsmann, O.: Asymmetrische Leukozytenbefunde bei Lungentuberkulose. Wr. Klin. Wschr. 77/37, 618 (1965).
–, –: Herdwirkung in der Pulmologie. Die Therapiewoche 15/24, 1284 (1965).
–, –, *Damböck, E.:* Venöse Oxy-Hämoglobin- und Leukozytenseitendifferenz unter Reizkörperbehandlung. Beitr. Klin. Tub. 139, 295–304 (1969).
–, –, *Kellner, G., Maresch, O.:* Synopse zur Frage der biologischen Regulationen. Ärztl. Praxis XXIII. 933, 1061, 1193, 1376 (1971).
–, –: Tuberkulöse Lungenprozesse und Makroregulation. Reprint from Pneumonology Vol. 143 (1970) 247.
–, –: Durchströmungsasymmetrien der Subclaviaarterien in Abhängigkeit von Lungenprozessen. Wien Z. f. Inn. Med. u. ihre Grenzgeb. 52 (1972) 152.
–, –: Abkühlungstests in der Thermodiagnostik. Phys. Ther. u. Rehab. 21 (1980) 661.
–, –: weiteres: siehe Beitrag *Bergsmann.*
v. Bertalanffy: 1952: zit. nach *H. Heine,* Die Grundregulation aus neuer Sicht. ÄZ. f. NHVerf. 28 (1987) 909.
Bessis, M.: Cellules du sang. Masson et Cie 1972.
Bethe, A.: Allgemeine Physiologie. Springer-Verlag Berlin-Heidelberg 1952.
Bethge, H.: Alternierende Corticoid-Therapie. Dt. Med. WS 96 (1971) 1254.
Biermann, H. K., Kelly, Petrakis, Cordes, Forster, Lose: The effect of intraven. histamin administration on the level of the white blood count in the peripheral blood. Blood 6, 926 (1951).
Bircher, F. E.: Autoallergie. Ott-Verlag 1968.
Birkmeier, W. und *Winkler, W.:* Klinik und Therapie der vegetativen Funktionsstörung. Wien, Springer-Verlag (1951).
Boeke, J.: The sympath. endformation, its synaptology, the interstitial cells, the periterminal network and its bearing on the neurone theory. Discussion and critique. Acta anatm. (Basel). 8, 18 (1949).
Bogomolez, H.: Konstitution und Mesenchym. Ref. Zentralbl. f. allg. Pathol. und pathol. Anat. 35, 375, 1924/25.
Bordeu, L.: Recherches sur le tissu muqueux ou l'organ cellulaire. Paris 1767, 1 und 2.
Botar, J.: Physiologisch-morphologische Untersuchungen über die Innervation des Nebennierenmarkes beim Hund. Acta. anat. 35, Suppl. 33, 1–88 (1958).
–, –: The innervation of the heart musculature and its changes. Z. mikr. anat. Forsch. 70, 168–214 (1963).
Brettschneider, H.: Die Gefäßinnervation als ein Beispiel für die feinere Morphologie der veget. Endformation. Anat. Anz. 113, 150–171 (1964).
Brückle, G.: Beobachtungen an der terminalen Unterlippenschleimhaut des Menschen unter besonderer Berücksichtigung der funktionellen Reaktionen. Vortrag am Int. Kongreß f. Herdforschg. Baden bei Wien, 1969.

–, –: Kapillarmikroskopische Untersuchungen über die Wirkung eines Glyko-Peptid-Komplexes auf die geschädigte Gefäßwand. Die Medizin. Welt 41, 1–19 (1969).

Bucher, O.: Cytologie, Histologie und mikroskopische Anatomie d. Menschen. Verl. Hans Huber, Bern, Stuttgart, Wien, 1970.

Busch, H. J. und *Busch, L.:* Abschlußbericht über Forschungsauftrag d. BM f. Verteidigung, BRD vom 30. 11. 1969.

–, –, *Busch, L.:* Mitteilung bei der 30. Jahrestagung der Dt. Arb. Gem. für Herd- u. Regul. Frschg. Bad Nauheim 1979.

Buttersack, F.: Latente Erkrankungen des Grundgewebes, insbesondere der serösen Häute. Stuttgart (1912).

Cajal, Ramon S.: Sur les ganglions et plexus nerveux de l'intestin. C. R. Soc. Biol. V/39, 217 (1893/94).

Carere-Comes, O.: Über die menschlichen bluthaltigen Lymphknoten. Folia hämat. 59, (1938).

Carrel, A. und *Ebeling, A. H.:* J. exp. med. Vol. 44 Nr. 2, 261, 261 (1926). J. of exp. Medicine, 44, Nr. 3, 285 (1926).

Chwalla und Keibl: zitiert nach *Eppinger* „Permeabilitätspathologie".

Croon, R.: Elektroneural-Diagnostik und Therapie nach Croon. Physik. Med. und Rehabil. Jg. 17/44, 81 (1976).

Diehl, F.: Studien zur Permeabilität der menschlichen Haut unter verschiedenen Bedingungen. Z. f. exp. Med. 100, 145–191 (1937).

Dosch, J. P.: Lehrbuch der Neuraltherapie nach Huneke (Procain-Therapie), 12. Aufl. 1986. Dort weitere Literatur.

Eberius, E.: Wasserbestimmung mit Karl Fischer-Lösung. Verl. Chemie, Weinheim (1958).

Ehinger, B.: Distribution of adrenergic nerves in the eye and some related structures in the cat. Acta physiol. scand 66, 123 (1966).

Ehrlich, P.: Das Sauerstoffbedürfnis des Organismus. Eine farbenanalytische Studie. Berlin 1885.

Eppinger, H.: Die Permeabilitätspathologie als die Lehre vom Krankheitsbeginn. Springer-Verlag Wien (1949).

Falck, B.: Observations of the cellular localisation of monoamines by a fluorescence method. Acta physiol. Scnad. 56, Suppl. 197, 1–25 (1962).

Feyrter, F.: Über die Pathologie der vegetativen nervösen Peripherie und ihrer ganglionären Regulationsstätten. Verl. W. Maudrich, Wien 1951.

Filatow, W. P.: Die biologischen Grundlagen der Gewebstherapie. Sowjetwissenschaft, naturw. Abtg. 1, 37–76 (1952).

Fleckenstein, A.: Die periphere Schmerzauslösung und Schmerzausschaltung. Steinkopff, Frankfurt 1950.

–, –: Bioelektrische und biochemische Primärreaktionen bei der Entzündungsgenese. In „Herderkrankungen Grundlagenforschung und Praxis". Carl Hanser München, 1956.

Foulk und *Bauden:* J. Am. chem. Soc. 48, 2045 (1926).

Freund, F. und *Kaminer, G.:* Biochemische Grundlagen der Disposition für Carcinom. Springer-Verlag, Wien 1925.

Fudalla, S. G.: Zur Biologie des Mesenchyms. Synopt. Versuch etc. Hippokr. 26, 23/24, 693–697, 740–744 (1955).

–, –: Das Herdgeschehen im Wandel der Zeiten. Physik. Med. und Rehab. Jg. 16/19, 190–194 (1975).

Gabler, E. und *Bejdl, W.:* Die Allergie der Albinoratten unter Kalbserum-Antigen-Einwirkung. Z. Immun- und Allergieforsch. **127**, 184–194 (1964).

Gerlach, F.: Biologie der Mykoplasmen und ihre Beziehung zu malignen Tumoren. Wien. Tierärztl. Monatsschr. **57**, 232–245 (1970).

Gerson, M.: Eine Krebstherapie. Bericht über 50 geheilte Fälle. Hyperion-Verlag, Freiburg/Br. 1958.

Gibian, H.: Beitrag des Chemikers zur Struktur und Funktionsaufklärung der mesenchymalen Grundsubstanz usw. in „Kapillaren und Interstitium", hrsg. von H. Bartelheimer und Kuchmeister; G. Thieme-Verlag, Stuttgart 1955.

Gildemeister, F.: Über elektrischen Widerstand, Kapazität und Polarisation der Haut. II. Mitt. Pflügers Arch. f. ges. Phys. **219**, 98–110 (1928).

Häbler, C.: Physikochemische Medizin nach H. Schade. Steinkopf, Dresden (1939).

Hauss, W. H.: Über die Entstehung und Behandlung rheumatischer Erkrankungen. Hippokrates **32/17**, 678 (1961).

–, –, *Junge-Hülsing, G.:* Über die universelle unspezifische Mesenchymreaktion. Dtsch. med. Wschr. **86/16**, 763–768 (1961).

Hauswirth, O.: Vegetative Konstitutionstherapie. Springer-Verlag, Wien 1953.

–, –: Bioklimatologie und Klimatherapie, Physiotherapie 64. Jg. Lübeck, März 1973, H. 3.

–, –: Die D'Arsonvalisation oder Zeileistherapie. Der deutsche Badebetrieb, Jg. **62**, 1–8 (1971).

Havlicek, H.: zitiert bei *Sehrt, E.:* Elektive ultraviolette Strahlung etc. Siehe unter *Sehrt*.

Heine, H.: Der Extrazellulärraum – eine vernachlässigte Dimension der Tumorforschung. Krebsgeschehen 17 (1985) 124.

–, –: Weitreichende Wechselwirkung als Grundlage der Homöostase – funktionelle Aspekte der Neuraltherapie. ÄZ f. NHVerf. 28 (1987) 915.

–, –: Die Grundregulation aus neuer Sicht. ÄZ f. NHVerf. 28 (1987) 909.

–, –, *Schaeg, G.:* Informationssteuerung in der vegetativen Peripherie. Z. f. Hautkrh. 54 (1979) 590.

Hertting, G. und *Suko, J.:* Influence of Neuronal and Extraneuronal Uptake on Disposition, Metabolism, and Potency of Catecholamines. Perspectives in Pharmacology, a Tribute to Jul. Axelrod. Oxford University Press Inc. 1972.

Hertwig, O.: Die Entwicklung des mittleren Keimblattes der Wirbeltiere. Jena 1881/82.

Hess, R. W.: Funktionelle Organisation des vegetativen Nervensystems. B. Schwabe Verlag, Basel 1948.

–, –: Das Zwischenhirn, Syndrome, Lokalisationen, Funktionen. B. Schwabe-Verlag, Basel 1949.

Höber, R.: Lehrbuch der Physiologie des Menschen. Springer-Verlag, Berlin, 1920.

–, –: Physikalische Chemie der Zellen und Gewebe. Stämpfli-Bern (1947).

Hoff, F.: Klinische Physiologie und Pathologie. G. Thieme-Verlag, Stuttgart, 1962.

Holasek und *Winsauer:* pers. Mittlg. Zit. b. Pischinger, A. 1957.

Horstmann, E.: Lymphgefäßbewegungen. Farbtonfilm, Kiel: Inst. wiss. Film Göttingen, 1958.

Huek, W.: Zieglers, Beitr. z. pathol. Anat. u. z. allg. Pathol, **66**, 330 (1920).

–, –: Münchn. med. Wochenschr. Nr. **19**, 535 (1920).

–, –: Münchn. med. Wochenschr. **20**, 573 (1920).

–, –: Münchn. med. Wochenschr. **21**, 606 (1920).

–, –: Münchn. med. Wochenschr. **37**, 1325 (1922).

–, –: Das Mesenchym. Naturwissensch. **141**, (1923).

Humphrey, J. H., Withe, R. G.: Kurzes Lehrbuch der Immunologie, 2. Aufl. Verlag G. Thieme, Stuttgart 1972.
Huneke, F.: Das Sekunden-Phänomen. 5., verb. Aufl. 1983, Karl F. Haug Verlag, Heidelberg.
Ito, Toshio: Recent advances in the study on the fine structure of the hepatic sinusoidal wall: a review. Gunma Rep. Med. Sci. 6, 119–163 (1973).
Jabonero, V.: Die vegetative Peripherie. Acta neurovegetat. (Wien) Suppl. IV (1955).
–, –: Studien über die Synapsen des peripheren vegetativen Nervensystems. Acta neurovegetat. (Wien) 29/1, 111 (1966).
–, –, *Genis, M. S., Santos, L.:* Beobachtungen über die cadmiumzinkjodidaffinen Elemente der Vorsteherdrüse. Z. mikr. anat. Forsch. 69, 167–199 (1963).
Junge-Hülsing: Untersuchungen zur Pathophysiologie des Bindegewebes. Dr. A. Hüthig Verlag, Heidelberg 1965.
Kaiser, E.: Zellatmungsversuch in: Pischinger, Österr. Zschr. Stomat. 60, 294 (1963).
–, – u. *Stockinger, L.:* Morphologie u. Biochemie des Bindegewebes. Münch. Med. Wochenschr. 113/10, 321–333 (1971).
Kaufmann, H. P. und *Budwig, H.:* Fette und Seifen. 1952.
Keller, R.: Die Elektrizität in der Zelle. Jul. Kittls Nachfolger Keller u. Co., Mähr. Ostrau 1925.
Kellner, G.: Die Lymphwege der menschlichen Milz. Z. mikr.-anat. Forsch. 68, 564 (1962).
–, –: Die Wirkung des Herdes auf die Labilität des humoralen Systems. Österr. Z. Stomatol. 60, 312 (1963).
–, –: Nachweis der Herderkrankung und ihre Grundlagen. Die Therapiewoche 15/24, 1267 (1965).
–, –: Funktionelle Morphologie der Haut und der Narbe. Ärztl. Praxis 18, 89 und 105 (1966).
–, –: Physikochemische Phänomene bei der Metallimprägnation. Acta histochem. Suppl. X, 279–285 (1969).
–, –: Probleme der Wundsetzung und der beeinflußten Wundheilung. Österr. Zschr. f. Stomatol. 66, 122 (1969).
–, –: Herdgeschehen und Herdnachweis. ZWR 1 (1971).
–, –: Zum Konnex von Wundsetzung, Wundheilungsstörung und chronischer Entzündung. Österr. Zeitschr. f. Stomatol. 70, 82–89 (1973).
–, –, Klenkhart, E.: Zur Differenzierung der Serumjodometrie nach A. Pischinger (Elektrometrische Titration). Österr. Zeitschr. f. Erforschg. u. Bekämpfung der Krebskrankheit 25, 81–88 (1970).
–, –: Zur Histopathologie des Störfeldes am Beispiel der Narbe. Phys. Med. u. Rehab. 10 (1969) 4.
–, –: Wundheilung und Wundheilungsstörung. Erfahrungsheilkunde 20 (1971) 173.
–, –: Homöopathie als Arzneimittelreiztherapie. Öst. Apotheker-Ztg. 34 (1980) 272.
–, –, *Michalica, W., Picha, E.* und *Placheta, P.:* Versuche zur Verminderung der Belastung weiblicher Tumorkranker durch Strahlenbehandlung. Z. f. Erforsch. u. Bekämpfung d. Krebskrankheit 26, 180–191 (1971).
–, –, *Stacher, A.* und *Undt, W.:* Beiträge zur Medizin-Meteorologie 1. Grundsätzliches zur Korrelation von Wetter und Mensch. Z. angew. Bäder- u. Klimaheilk. 11, 1–4 (1964).
–, –, –, –, –: Aus der Bioklimatologie: Zur quantitativen Auswertung von Wettereinflüssen auf den Menschen. Med. Mitt. – Med. wiss. Abtlg. Schering AG-Berlin – 25, 23–29 (1964).

Kerjaschki, D. und *Stockinger, L.:* Struktur und Funktion des Perineuriums. Die Endigungsweise des Perineuriums vegetativer Nerv. n. Z. Zellforsch. **110**, 386–400 (1970).
Kerl, W.: Wien. Kl. WS. (1930), 1365 u. Derm. Wiss. 95 (1932), 1253. zit. n. *E. Urbach,* Klinik u. Ther. d. allerg. Krankheiten (1935).
Kern, B.: Der Myokardinfarkt. Karl F. Haug Verlag, Heidelberg 1974.
Kihara, T.: Das extravaskuläre Saftbahnsystem. Fol. Anat. Jap. **28**, 601 (1956).
Klingenberg, H. G.: Untersuchungen über die Wirkung elektrisch geladener Stoffe auf die glatte Muskulatur. Z. f. Biologie **108**, 312–320 (1956).
–, –,*Peters, E.:* Der Übertritt von Eiweiß und Wasser ins Gewebe unter physiologischen Verhältnissen. Wien. Z. Inn. Med. **30**, 22 (1949).
Koch, E.: Über leukozytäre Abbauzellen. Klin. Wschr. **29**, 474 (1951).
Koch, F. W.: Das Überleben bei Krebs und Viruskrankheiten. Das Schlüsselprinzip ihrer Heilbarkeit. Karl F. Haug Verlag, Heidelberg 1975.
Köhler, U.: Die perorale Strophanthintherapie der Angina pectoris. Notabene medici, 6. Jg., H. 8, Sonderdruck (August 1976).
Kohout, J.: Untersuchungen zur Immunreaktion vom Spättyp bei Erkrankungen der Lunge: Praxis der Pneumologie etc. **25**/9, 540 (1971).
–, –: Der Lymphozyt, Struktur etc. 1. Tagg.-Bericht d. Österr. Gesellsch. f. Hämatologie.
Kolb, R.: Nachweis von Katecholaminen in den Nerven der Pulmonalisklappe des Meerschweinchens. Acta neurovegetat. **29**/4, 579 (1967).
–, –, *Pischinger, A., Stockinger, L.:* Ultrastruktur der Pulmonalisklappe des Meerschweinchens: Beitrag zum Studium der vegetativ-nervösen Peripherie. Z. mikr.-anat. Forsch. **76**, 184 (1967).
Kölliker, A.: Mikroskopische Anatomie oder Gewebelehre des Menschen. Leipzig 1850.
–,–: Handbuch der Gewebelehre des Menschen. Leipzig 1889/1902.
Komiyra, E. und Mitarbeiter: Extraktion der neurohumoralen blutregulierenden Wirkstoffe. 2. Mitt. Extraktion von Monopoetin etc. Folia haematol. Neue Folge **5**, 328–348 (1961).
Kracmar, F.: Vegetative Konstitution und elektrischer Unfall. Elektromed. **6**, 169–174 (1961).
–, –: Über die Änderung des Polarisationswiderstandes und der Polarisationskapazität des menschlichen Körpers durch vegetative Pharmaka. Elektromed. **6**, 158–159 (1961).
–, –: Zur Biophysik des vegetativen Grundsystems. Physik. Medizin und Rehabilitation. Z. allg. Med. **12**, 120–122 (1971). Dort weitere Literatur.
Kraus, F.: Vegetatives System und Individualität. Dtsch. Med. Wochenschr. **48**, 1627 (1922).
Kraus, H.: Zur Morphologie, Systematik und Funktion der Lymphgefäße. Z. f. Zellforsch. **46**, 446–456 (1957).
–, –: Besonderheit der Kreislaufsteuerung im (lympho)-retikulären Bindegewebe gegenüber der Kreislaufsteuerung im kollagenen Bindegewebe. Anat. Anz. **109**, 225–230 (1961).
Krehl, S. und *Marchand, F.:* Handbuch der allgemeinen Pathologie. IV/Abt. 1, 1924, „Lehre von den Entzündung".
Krogh, A.: Die Anatomie und Physiologie der Kapillaren, Berlin, 1929.
Kunz, H. und *Popper, L.:* Zur Frage des Bakterienübertrittes aus der Blutbahn in die Lymphe. Z. Klin. Med. **128**, 568–582 (1935).
Lampert, H.: Die Bedeutung der Überwärmung für Klinik und Praxis. Ärztl. Praxis XIV/ 37, 1905/1921/1923 (1962).
Langley, J. N.: La systeme nerveux autonome. Vigot Paris 1923.

McLaughlin, C.B.: Symp. Soc. Exper. Biology 17, Cambridge 1963; zit. n. *F.M. Lehmann,* Biologie – Nr. 24 der Schr.-Reihe der Bez.Ärztekammer Nordwürttemberg, Verl. Gertner, Stuttgart 1976.

Laves, W.: Über Faktoren der Leukozytolyse. Schweiz. Med. Wschr. **84**/39, 1097 (1954).

Lawrentiew, B.J.: Über die Erscheinung der Degeneration und Regeneration im sympathischen Nervensystem. Z. mikr.-anat. Forsch. **2**, 201 (1925).

Leak, L.V.: Lymphatic capillaries in tail fin of Amphibian Larva: An electron microscopic study. Journ. Morphol. **125**/4, 419 (1968).

Leder, L.D.: Der Blutmonozyt. Springer-Verlag, Berlin-Heidelberg, New York, 1967.

Lennert, H.: Lymphknoten und Diagnostik; Bandteil A: Cytologie und Lymphadenitis. Handbuch d. spez. pathol. Anatomie und Histologie, Bd. I, Teil III, Springer-Verlag 1961.

Letterer, E.: Allgemeine Pathologie, Grundlagen und Probleme. G. Thieme, Stuttgart, 1959.

Leupold, E.: Der Zell- und Gewebsstoffwechsel als innere Krankheitsbedingung. G. Thieme-Verlag, Leipzig 1945 (I).

–, –: Die Bedeutung des Blutchemismus besonders in Beziehung zu Tumorbildung und Tumorabbau. II. Teil. G. Thieme Verlag, Stuttgart 1954.

Lickint, F.: Die Leukozytenreaktion nach der modernen Reiztherapie usw. Inaug. Diss. Leipzig (1923).

Lipp, W.: Studien zur Herzinnervation. Acta anat. **13**, 30 (1951).

–, –, *Rodin, M.:* Die adrenergen Nervenplexus in Herzklappen. Verh. d. Anat. Ges. 1967, 121/Erg. 83 (1968).

Löwenstein, W.R.: Permeability of Membrane junction. Ann. N.Y. Acad. Sci. **137**, 441–472 (1966).

Lumière: Grundlagen einer neuen Humanmedizin, Verlag für Medizin, Leipzig, 1927.

Lutz, F. und *Pischinger, A.:* Über einen neuen Faktor im tierischen Blut usw. Wien. Med. Wschr. 99 (1949), 437.

Maehder, K.: Über den Nachweis der perlingualen Strophanthin-Resorption mittels Isotopen. Med. Klinik 50. Jg. Nr. 2, 104–105 (1955).

Maillet, H.: Modifications de la technique de Champy au tetraoxyd l'osmiumiodide de Potassium. Results de son application à l'etude des fibres nerveuses. C.R. Soc. Biol. (Paris) **153**, 939 (1959).

Maresch, O.: Physikalische Beurteilung der Heilwässer. Vortrag Symposium über Bädertherapie. Mai 1970 in Baden-Wien.

Maruna, R.F.L., Gründig, E.: Wien. Med. Wschr. **117**, 903 (1967); Wien. Med. Wschr. **118**, 724 (1968).

–, –, *Stipinovic, G.:* Über den Bleigehalt der Oberschenkelknochen von Unfallpatienten im Raume Wien. Wien. Med. WS 124 (1974) 616.

McMaster u. *Hudack:* J. exp. Med. 61 (1935) 783.

Maximow, A.: Bindegewebe und blutbildendes Gewebe. In: Handbuch d. mikroskop. Anat. d. Menschen Bd. II/1, 232–583, Springer-Verlag, Berlin 1927.

Meier, A. und *Gottlieb, H.:* Experimentelle Pharmakologie. 8. Aufl. Urban und Schwarzenberg, 1933.

Meier-Synek, B.: Das vegetative System unter Kontrolle der Blut-Redox-Reaktion. Z. Kinderheilk. **63**/6, 711 (1943).

Metschnikoff, E.: Die Lehre von den Phagozyten und deren experimentelle Grundlagen. Handb. d. pathog. Mikroorganismen. W. Kolle und A. v. Wassermann, G. Fischer Jena, 1913.

Meyling, H. E.: Das periphere Nervennetz und sein Zusammenhang mit den ortho- und parasympathischen Nervenfasern. Acta neuroveg. Suppl. IV: Die neurovegetative Peripherie, 38–63; Springer-Verlag Wien, 1955.

Molenaar, H. und *Roller, D.:* Die Bestimmung des extrazellularen Wassers beim Gesunden und Kranken. Z. klin. Med. **136,** 1 (1939).

Möllendorff, W. von: Handbuch der mikr. Anat. d. Menschen, Bd. II, Berlin 1927.

–, –: Lehrbuch der Histologie und mikr. Anatomie d. Menschen. G. Fischer, Jena 1943.

Müller, L. R.: Die Lebensnerven. Berlin, 1931.

Nägeli: Zitiert bei *Leder* (1967).

Neuberger, F.: Zur Objektivierung endo- und exogener Einflüsse auf den Tonus des veget. Nervensystems. Acta oto-laryngol. **51,** 332–346.

Neuberger, F.: Zur Objektivierung endo- und exogener Einflüsse auf den Tonus der akustischen und/oder vestibularen Sensorik. Monatsschr. f. Ohrenheilkunde und Laryngo-Rhinologie **94,** 262–274 (1960).

Neuraltherapie nach Huneke: Freudenstädter Vorträge 1971/72. Herausgegeben von *J. P. Dosch,* Karl F. Haug Verlag, Heidelberg 1974.

Pape, R.: Ergebnisse und Fragen der Röntgen-Schwachbestrahlung. Strahlentherapie, Sonderband **35,** 116 (37. Jgg. München).

Perger, F.: Untersuchungen über den Wirkungsmechanismus der hochmolekularen Fettsäuren im Elpimed bei parenteraler Zuführung. Med. Klin. 51/31, 1299 (1956).

–, –: Die Elpimedreaktion zur Erfassung der vegetativen Grundsituation mittels der Blutkriterienbestimmung als Ganzheitstest. Österr. Z. f. Stomat. 60/11, 440 (1963).

–, –: Problematik der medikamentösen Therapie bei Herderkrankungen. Ärztl. Praxis XV/47, 2596 (1963).

–, –: Die Bedeutung der Grundregulation. Die therapeutischen Konsequenzen der Grundregulation. Erfahrungsheilkunde XXI, H. 9/11, 261–350 (1972).

–, –: Erfahrungsheilkunde **30,** 39 (1981).

–,–: Über den derzeitigen Stand der Herdforschung. EHK d. **26,** 140 (1977).

–, –: Chronische Entzündung und Carcinom aus der Sicht des Grundsystems. Wien. Med. WS **128,** 31 (1978).

–,–: Multiple Sklerose und Herdgeschehen. Wien. med. WS **126,** 283 (1976).

–, –: Öst. Zschr. f. Stomatologie **60,** 440 (1963).

–, –: Die Bestimmung der vegetativen Reaktionslage und Reaktionsweise bei Multiple Sklerose-Kranken. Dt. Med. WS. **81,** 342 (1956), (Allergiebeilage).

–, –: Herdtherapie – Erfolg und Mißerfolg. EHKd. **27,** 805 (1978).

–, –: Extranervale Steuerungsmechanismen. DZA **24,** 81 (1981).

–, –: Sinn und Unsinn von Herdsanierungen bei Erkrankungen des rheumatischen Formenkreises. Rheuma **4,** 1 (1981).

–, –: Immunstimulation über das Grundsystem mit körpereigenen Stoffen. EHKd. **35,** 146 (1986).

–, –: Regulationsstörungen und Darmkeimverhältnisse. EHKd. **34,** 812 (1985).

–, –: Klinische Aspekte des Zinkmangels beim Menschen. D. prakt. Arzt **40,** 1591 (1986).

–, –: Die Vor- und Nachbehandlung von Herdsanierungen. Neuramed **2,** 12 und 68 (1987).

–, –: Das Zusammenspiel zwischen den Regelsystemen der Abwehr und seine Störungen. EHKd. **36,** 566 (1987).

–, –: Unterschiedliche Entwicklung der Schwermetallbelastungen (Pb, Cd, Hg) und ihre Therapie. Z. f. NHVerf. **28**, 774 (1987).

–, –: Fragen der Herderkrankung. D. Zahnärztekal. 1988, S. 23–38, Verlag C. Hanser, München 1988.

–, –: Klinik der Lambliasis intestinalis und ihre Verbreitung in Mitteleuropa. Naturamed **3** (1988), Heft 1.

Perger F., Maruna R.: Zur Frage der subsymptomatischen Schwermetallbelastung beim Menschen (Pb Cd, Hg). EHKd. **35**, 316 (1986).

–, –: Ergebnisse von Blut-, Harn- und Haaranalysen auf Schwermetalle. Dt. Z. f. biolog. Zahnmed. **3**, 107 (1987).

Petersen, H.: Über Methoden zum Studium des Knochens. Z. wiss. Mikr. **43**, 355 (1926).

Petueli, R.: Biochemische Untersuchungen zur Regulation der Dickdarmflora des Säuglings. Verlag Notring der wissenschaftl. Verbände Österr., Wien 1957.

Pfeiffer, H.: Wien. Klin. Wochenschr. **30**, 363 (1921).

–, –, *Standenath, Fr.:* Z. f. d. ges. exp. Med. **37**, 184.

Pichlmayr, R. und Mitarb.: Gewinnung von heterologen Immunseren gegen menschliche Lymphozyten. Klin. Wschr. **46**, 249–258 (1968).

Pischinger, A.: Die Lage des isoelektrischen Punktes histologischer Elemente als Ursache ihrer verschiedenen Färbbarkeit. Z. Zellf. u. mikr. Anat. **3** (1926).

–, –: Neue Beobachtungen zur Aufklärung der Moorwirkung. Die österr. Moorforschg. **4**, (1953).

–, –: Schicksal und Wirkung körperfremden Gewebes im Organismus. Die Medizinische, **23**, 6. 6. 1953.

–, –: Pathologische Grundlagen und Probleme der Herderkrankungen. Nauheimer Tagung der DAH. Hanser Verlag, München 1954.

–, –: Untersuchungen am Blute nach künstlicher Oxygenation. Münchn. Med. Wschr. **96**, 879 (1954).

–, –: Das System des Unspezifischen und seine Bedeutung für das Herdgeschehen. In: Herderkrankungen, Grundlagenforschung und Praxis. Hanser Verlag, München 1956.

–, –: Neue Auffassungen über das Vegetativum, seine Organisation und Bedeutung für das Herdgeschehen. Österr. Z. Stomatologie **53**, 621–629 (1956).

–, –: Die Bedeutung hochmolekularer ungesättigter Fettsäuren im Blut. Therapiewoche **7**, 397 (1957).

–, –: Das Schicksal der Leukozyten. Z. mikr.-anat. Forsch. **63**, 169–192 (1957).

–, –: Über die Zellen des weichen Bindegewebes. Wien. Kl. Wschr. **71** 73–77 (1959).

–, –: Über die vegetativen, insbesondere humoralen Grundlagen des Herdgeschehens. Ärztl. Praxis XIII, 249–251 (1961).

–, –: Der Monozyt des Blutes. Symp. Biol. Hung. Vol. **2**, 27–36 (1961).

–, –: Über die Organisation des lymphatischen Gewebes. Z. Zellforsch. **60**, 893 bis 908 (1963).

–, –: Die Objektivierung des Sekundenphänomens (*F. Huneke*). Physikalisch-Diätetische Therapie **6**, 1–6 (1965).

–, –: Aussprache zu *Humplick, H.:* Cephalea-frontalis-Galeatomie. (Vortrag) Wien. Klin. Wschr. **77**, 912 (1965).

–, –: Krebs und Abwehreinrichtungen des Organismus. Hier mit *G. Draczynski* und *G. Kellner:* Serumjodometrie. Krebsarzt **21**, 297–311 (1966).

–, –: Zur Grundlegung unspezifischer Behandlungsweisen. Physikalische Medizin und Rehabilitation **9**, 7–12 (1968).

–, –: Über das vegetative Grundsystem. Physikalische Med. und Rehabilitation 10, 53–57 (1969).

–, –: Die Grundregulation. Erfahrungsheilkunde 10, 301. 363. 11 (1971/72).

–, –: Erfahrungsheilkunde 28, 317 (1979).

–, –: Objektivierbarkeit der Neuraltherapie mittels Serumjodometrie sowie elektrische Messungen. Frühj. Symposium 1974 d. Österr. Gesellschaft f. Neuraltherapie (Fieberbrunn) (GEBRO).

–, –: Das Konzept des „Ganzheitssystems" als Weg zum Verständnis der Neuraltherapie. Die ärztliche Fortbildung 1, 27–30 (1975).

–, –: Die humoral-zelluläre Reaktion des lympho-monozytären Systems. EHKd. 28, 317 (1979).

–, –, *Stockinger, L.:* Die Nerven der menschlichen Zahnpulpa. Z. Zellforsch. 89, 44–61 (1968).

Plenk, H. jr. und *Raab, H.:* Die Nerven der menschlichen Gingiva. Z. mikr.-anat. Forsch. 81, 153–181 (1969).

–, –, –, –: Die Nerven der menschlichen Gingiva (II. Mitteilung: Weitere histochemische und elektronenmikroskopische Befunde). Z. mikr.-anat. Forsch. 81, 473–491 (1970).

Plohberger, H. M.: Karzinom und Herdgeschehen. Österr. Z. f. Erforschg. und Bekämpfung der Krebskrankheit. 27. Jg. H. 3, 63–69 (1972).

Plohberger, R. und *Kracmar, F.:* Krebsbehandlung nach Prof. Leupold im Spiegel der Biophysik. Erfahrhk. 19, 458 (1970).

–, –, –, –: Krebsbehandlung nach Professor *Leupold* im Spiegel der Biophysik. Krebsgeschehen, 111–118 (1971).

Popp, F. A.: Biophotonen. Schriftenreihe Krebsgeschehen Bd. 6, 2. Aufl. VfM Dr. Ewald Fischer, Heidelberg 1984.

Raab, H.: Die klinische Bedeutung des Nachweises von adrenergen, autonomen Nerven im menschlichen Zahnfleisch. Österr. Z. Stomat. 67, 381–390 (1970).

–, –: Die vegetativen Grundlagen dentogener Herderkrankungen. W. Maudrich, Wien 1972.

Ratzenhofer, M.: Morphologie und Bedeutung der Funktionsstörung des Mesenchyms nebst Beobachtungen über Veränderungen am Gefäß-Nervengewebe beim Karzinom. Wien. Med. Wschr. 100, 646–652 (1950).

–, –: Innervationsstudien am Magen. 10. Tagg. der Österr. Gesellsch. f. Chirurgie, 26–28. 6. 1969, Graz.

–, –: Vorkommen und Bedeutung freier Gewebsflüssigkeit in der weiblichen Brustdrüse.

–, –, *Klingenberg, H. G.* und *Schauenstein, E.:* Zur Histologie der Gewebsflüssigkeit und über ihren Gehalt an Eiweiß und aromatischen Aminosäuren. I. Mitteilung.

–, –, *Schauenstein, E.:* Über den Nachweis von Albuminen im Gewebssaft bei krebsig entarteter Mastopathien.

Rebuck, J. W. und *Crowley, J. H.:* Ann. N. Y. Acad. Sci. 59, 757 (1955).

Reichert, C. B.: Vergleichende Beobachtungen über das Bindegewebe und die verwandten Gebilde. Dorpat 1845, S. 168.

Reinstorff, E.: Ein Beitrag zur Molekularmagnetik des Wassers Wetter-Boden-Mensch, Forschungskreis für Geobiologie e. V., H. 3.

Reiser, K. A.: Über die Innervation der Hornhaut des Auges. A. Augenheilk. 109, 251 (1935).

v. Riccobona, A.: Kritik der Herderkrankungen vom HNO-Arzt. In: Krit. Betrachtung des Herdgeschehens (DAH-Kongr. 1954), Verlag C. Hanser, München 1955.
eRicker, G.: Pathologie als Naturwissenschaft. Berlin 1925.
Rilling, S.: Binotonometrie, Grundlagen und Anwendungen. Stuttgart 1971.
v. Rindfleisch, E.: Elemente der Pathologie. Leipzig 1869.
Rockitansky, C. v.: Handbuch der pathologischen Anatomie. Wien 1846.
Rohr, K.: Blut- und Knochenmarksmorphologie der Agranulozyten (Ergebnisse fortlaufender Sternalmarkuntersuchungen). Fol. hämol. (Lpz.) 55, 305–367 (1936).
Rothmund, W.: Neue Aspekte zur Infarktforschung. Ein Diskussionsbeitrag. Zeitschrift f. Allgemeinmedizin (ZfA) 52. Jg. H. 16, 952–960 (1976).
Rudich, A.: Probleme der oralen Strophanthinbehandlung. Physik. Med. und Rehabilitation, 13. Jg./7, 206–211 (1972).
–, –: Das menschliche Knochenmark. Georg Thieme-Verlag, Stuttgart 1960.
Ruhenstroth-Bauer, G., Fuhrmann, Bey, Hertel: Änderung der Membranladung von Rattenleberzellen usw. Klin. Wschr. 44/39 (1966).
Rumler, K.: Der Säure-Base-Haushalt im Rahmen der Gesetzmäßigkeit der biologischen Regulation. Ärztl. Praxis, XXIII Jg., S. 420; 481; 541 (1971).
–, –: Beeinflussung der Regulation durch Ernährung. Erf.hk. XX/9, 269–276 (1972).
Ruska, H. und *Ruska, C.:* Licht- und Elektronenmikroskopie des peripheren neurovegetativen Systems in Hinblick auf die Funktion. Dtsch. med. Wschr. 86/36, 37; 1967 und 1770 (1961).
Salzer, G.M., Stockinger, L.; Zenker, W.: Die Ultrastruktur des juxta-oralen Organs der Ratte. Z. Zellforsch. 62, 829–854 (1964).
Sarre, H.: Strophanthinbehandlung bei Angina pectoris. Die Therapiewoche. Ber. üb. d. ges. Therapie (III. Jg. 1952/53, 13/14, 311–314 (1953).
Sato, Itio: Studien über die Antigenität der monozytogenen Substanzen im Blut. J. Chosen med. Assoc. 29/11, Deutsche Zusammenfassung, 328–329 (1939) Japan.
Schabadasch: Intramurale Nervengeflechte des Darmrohres. Z. Zellforsch. 10, 320–385 (1930).
Schade, H.: Die physikalische Chemie in der inneren Medizin, 3. Aufl., 1912.
Schaffer, J.: Lehrbuch der Histologie und Histogenese. W. Engelmann, Leipzig 1922.
Schauenstein, E.: Österr. Chemiker-Zeitung 52, 28 (1951).
Schauenstein, E.: Pibus, B.: Nachweis von Lipo-Peroxyden im menschlichen Serum. Wr. Klin. Wschr. 68/19, 376 (1956).
–, –: Autoxydation of polyunsaturated esters in water: chemical structure and biological activity of the products. J. of Lipid Research, V. 8, 417–428 (1967).
Schilling, V.: Praktische Blutlehre. 8/9. Aufl., Jena 1938.
Schliephake, E.: Kurzwellentherapie. 5. Aufl. Piscator-Verlag, Stuttgart 1952.
Schoeler, H.: Über elektrische Widerstandsmessungen an biologischen Geweben insbesondere an der Haut. Tggs-Bericht, Freudenstadt d. intern. Gesellsch. f. Neuraltherapie n. Huneke, 91–101 (1960).
Schöffler, H. H.: Zur Ätiologie des Herzinfarkts. Erf.hk., 1976/H 1, 6 (1976).
Schröder, H. J.: Gesetzmäßigkeiten bei der Nekrobiose und Autolyse der weißen Blutzellen und ihre biologische Bedeutung. Habil.-Schr. Med. Fak. d. Univ. Hamburg, 1959 (Hier weitere Literatur).
Schröder, H. und *Schröder, J.:* In vitro-Untersuchungen über die Wirkung des Zigarettenrauchens auf die Vitalität der Leukozyten. Fol. hämat. 87, 190–198 (1967).

Schröder, J.: Über gesetzmäßige Veränderungen der weißen Blutzellen in hypotoner Flüssigkeit. Z. Zellforsch. **46,** 300 (1957).

–, –: Der Einfluß blutchemischer Veränderungen auf die Fermentaktivität der Leukozyten. Acta hämat. **19,** 156, 1958.

Schröder, J.: Titerbestimmung der antilymphozyt. und der antigranulozyt. Wirkung des antilymphozyten-Immunserums (ALS) von *R. Pichlmayr* u. Mitarb. Beitr. z. gerichtl. Medizin, 316–319. Verl. Franz Deuticke, Wien 1970.

Schulze, W.: Untersuchungen über die Kapillaren und postkapillären Venen lymphatischer Organe. Z. Anat. Entwickl. Gesch. **76,** 421 (1925).

Schwamm, E.: Die Ultrarotabstrahlung und ihre medizinische Bedeutung. Erf.hk. **4,** 481–501 (1955).

Seeger, P.-G.: Vergleichende mikrochemische Untersuchungen an normalen Exsudatzellen und den Tumorzellen des Ehrlichschen Asziteskarzinoms der Maus. Der Kalium-Natriumkontrast. Z. f. mikr. anat. Forsch. **53,** 65–101 (1943).

Seelich, F. und *Stockinger, L.:* Ein Beitrag zum Problem der Zellform und deren Umwandlung. Z. Zellforsch. **39,** 212–231 (1953).

Seeling, W. et al.: Die Funktion des Zinks im Organismus – dargestellt am Beispiel der Akrodermatitis enteropatica. Med. Welt **28,** 1537 (NF 1977).

Sehrt, E.: Elektive Ultraviolettbestrahlung in Therapie und Prophylaxe. Hippokrates-Verlag Marquardt u. Cie. Stuttgart 1942: Kap. IV und V. Dort weitere Literatur über Havlicek.

Selye, H.: Einführung in die Lehre vom Adaptationssyndrom. G. Thieme, Stuttgart 1953.

Sieberth, E.: Blutchemische Veränderungen im Verlauf der Karzinomkrankheit. Fortschritte der Krebsforschung, Molekularbiol. etc. Bericht über die 10. wissensch. Tagg. des dtsch. Zentralausschusses für Krebsbek. und Krebsforschung e. V. Berlin 1968, S. 219 (dort weitere Literatur.)

Siegmund, H.: Speicherung durch Retikuloendothelien, zelluläre Reaktion und Immunität. Klin. Wschr. 1. Jg. **52,** S. 2566 (1922).

Sommer, H.: Erfahrungsbericht über Elpimed (früher Polyval) Med. Klinik **48,** 1224 (1952).

Speransky, A. D.: Grundlagen der Theorie der Medizin. Deutsch v. *K. P. von Roques.* Verlag Dr. W. Sänger, Berlin 1950.

Stacher, A.: Zur Wirkung der Herde auf den Gesamtorganismus. Österr. Zeitschr. f. Stomat. **63,** 294–303 (1966).

–, –: Über das Huneke-Sekundenphänomen und seine Objektivierung. In Voss Ferd. „Deshalb Neuraltherapie". Verl. Blume u. Co., s. 138–149.

Standenath, F.: Das Bindegewebe usw. Ergeb. d. allg. pathol. Anatomie d. Menschen u. d. Tiere 22, Abtlg. II 70.

Stern und *Willhelm:* Z. Krebsforsch. **46,** 379 (1937) zit. bei *Hinsberg*, Krebsproblem.

Stockinger, L.: Disse'scher Raum und Bindegewebszellen in der menschlichen Leber. Anat. Anz. Erg. H. zu **120,** 545–551 (1967).

–, –: Ultrastruktur und Histophysiologie der menschlichen Leber. Wr. Klin. Wschr. **81/23,** 431 (1969).

–, –: Morphologische Grundlagen der Erregungsübertragung in zellulären Systemen. Wissenschaft und Weltbild **25,** 73–87 (1972).

Stockinger, L. und *Pritz, W.:* Morphologische Aspekte der Schmerzempfindung im Zahn. Deutsch. Zahnärztl. Zeitschr. **25,** 357–363 (1970).

Stöhr, jr. Ph.: Mikroskopische Anatomie des vegetativen Nervensystems. Handb. d. mikr. Anat. d. Menschen v. Möllendorf-Bargmann, Bd. IV/5, Springer 1967.

Storck, H.: Rheumatismus als Regulationskrankheit. Verlag Urban und Schwarzenberg, München-Berlin 1954.
Undritz, E.: Über das Vorkommen von Abbauformen von Leukozyten im Blut. Fol. hämat. **65**, 195 (1941).
Undt, W., Karobath, H. u. Mitarb.: Der Herzmuskelinfarkt. Untersuchungen über den Einfluß von Wetter etc. auf den Zeitpunkt des Krankheitsbeginnes. Z. f. angew. Bäder- und Klimakunde **19**, 2/3 (1972).
Urbach, E.: Klinik und Therapie der allergischen Krankheiten. Verlag W. Maudrich, Wien 1935.
Virchow, R.: Die Cellularpathologie in ihrer Bedeutung auf physiologische und pathologische Gewebslehre. Hirschwald, Berlin 1858.
Voss, H. F.: Deshalb Neuraltherapie; 70 Arbeiten über die Neuraltherapie, ML-Verlag. Schriftenreihe des Zentralverbandes d. Ärzte für Naturheilverfahren, herausg. v. Dr. H. Haferkamp, Bd. 20.
Zabel, W.: Ganzheitsbehandlung der Geschwulsterkrankungen. Hippokrates, Verl. Marquardt u. Cie, Stuttgart.
–, –: Körpereigene Abwehr gegen Krebs. Med. Liter. Verlag, Hamburg.
Zen, Shomo: Studien über Monozytose durch Organextrakt, besonders über die Bedeutung des RES, welches diese Organe enthalten. J. Chosen med. Assoc. **30**, Nr. 1, dtsch. Zusammenfassung, 173–174 (1940).
Zischka, W.: Infektionskrankheiten. Verlag Urban und Schwarzenberg 1961.
Zypen, E. van der: Elektronenmikroskopische Befunde an der Endausbreitung des vegetativen Nervensystems und ihre Deutung. Acta anat. **67**, 431–515 (1967).

(Dr. med. Felix Perger, Kaiserstr. 123/9, A-1070 Wien)

Sachregister

A

α-chain 61
α-ketoglutarate 61
acidosis 202
ACTH 162
acupuncture 90, 98, 101, 113, 120, 124, 128, 132, 136
adaptation syndrome 88
adjustment arm 85
alarm reaction 146, 163
albumin 27, 28
allergies 175
allysine 66
amino acid 28
anesthesia 91
anthroposophic 78
antibiotics 175, 191
antigen 72
antigen protein 28
antioxidant systems 26
antishock 147
arteriovenous anastomoses 143
ascorbic acid 26, 61
asialoglycoprotein 49
asymmetry 93
asynchronism 93
AT-phosphatases 166, 195
ATP 26, 43, 169
autonomic nerves 132
autonomic regulation 182

B

bacteria 198
basement membrane 51, 63
basophilic granulocytes 47
biocybernetics 84, 88
biologically closed electric circuits (BCEC) 106
biophoton 52
biopolymers 46
bladder papilloma 173
blockade 152, 167, 168, 177
blood smears 39
blood-brain barrier 51
brain stem 159
bronchial asthma 91

C

CA^{2+} 51
calcium 183, 191
cAMP 26, 43, 48
cancer cells 183
capillary 20, 51, 112
carboxyhemoglobin 28
cartilage 56, 57
catalase 26
catecholamines 47
causal-analytical linearity 13
cell membrane 19, 27
cell pathology 9
cellular pathology 13
cellulose 77
cGMP 26, 48
cholesterin 28
cholesterol 155, 183
chondroitin sulfate 48, 56
chondronectin 69, 73
chronic diseases 9, 13, 56, 83, 90, 154
chronic inflammation 160
chronicity 89, 95
circadian rhythm 43
CNS 44, 45, 51, 159, 166
coagulation 72
coferment 160
Coli strains 176
collagen 19, 25, 27, 28, 58, 60
collagen fibril 59, 61
collagenase 62
complement factor C3 47
connective tissue 15, 16, 44
copper 160
corneal dystrophy 60
Coulombian charges 74
countershock 146
cyclic adenosine monophosphate 19
Cytochalasin A and B 70
cytokins 29, 31

D

D-galactose 60
D-glucouronic acid 46
D-penicillamin 66
decoder 127

217

dequi 115, 116
dermatan sulfate 56
dermatome system 125
desmosin 66
detoxification 194, 196
diaphragm 93, 115
diencephalon-hypothalamic control system 104
diet 185
disturbance field 90, 105, 159, 180, 181, 185
DNA 20, 24, 26, 61, 161
domain 52, 57
double refraction 65
dyspnea 115
dysregulation 9, 83, 92

E
E. coli 191
ECG 128
economy 84
eczema 175
edema 192
EEG 128
elastic fibers 68
elastin 19, 25, 27, 58
electrical polarization 64
electrolytes 147
electrons 24
electrotherapy 35
Elpimed 35, 155
EMG 128
endoplasmic reticulum 55
endothelial cells 72
energy flow 73
enthalpy 74, 75
entropy 68, 75
eosinophilic granulocytes 145
eosinophils 36
Eppstein-Barr virus 172
etheric body 78
etiology 94
eutectic point 53
expiration 92
extracellular matrix 14, 19, 20, 25, 26, 29, 31, 41, 42, 44, 45, 51, 52, 53, 58, 74, 75, 76, 113, 132, 158, 188
factor L 169
factor M 35, 141, 152, 153, 154
factor XIII 70
fascia 114

fatty acids 154
fibrinogen-complement 28
fibroblasts 34
fibrocytes 47
fibronectin 19, 25, 47, 49, 58, 69, 71, 72, 73
focal disease 88
foci 91, 105, 185
focus 159
formatio reticularis 99

F
Freund-Kaminer's cytolysis 39
fucose 69
fungi 173, 176, 177, 197

G
α-glucosamine 59
G proteins 48
GAGs 45, 46, 48, 58, 61
galactosamine 59
galactose 69
Galen 17
Galilei 13
gate control 96
gel 111
Giordano Bruno 78
globulins 170
glucose 185
glutathion peroxidase 26
glycine 61
glycocalyx 14, 48, 49
glycoprotein 28, 69
glycosaminoglycans 19
glycosylation 60
Goethe 78
granulocytes 165
ground regulation 7, 8, 148, 163, 190
ground system 104, 108, 120, 121, 136, 163, 164, 168, 178, 182, 192, 202

H
Hahnemann 17, 76
HbA_{1c} 27
Heine cylinder 106, 111
helix formation 61
hematogenous oxidation 186
hemograms 145
heparan sulfate 48, 59
heparin 46, 47
hexosamines 45
Hippocrates 17

homeopathic methods   17
homeopathy   76
homeostasis   30, 84, 128
humoral factors   15
Huneke's phenomenon   178, 179, 181
hyaluronic acid   25, 46, 48, 57
hydrolytic enzymes   29
hydrotherapy   35
hydroxylapatite   62
hydroxylysine   61
hydroxyproline   61
hypercholesterinemia   28
hypertonicity   124
hypothalamus   104
hysteresis   119

I
IgA   171
IgG   161, 171
IgM   171
immune processes   154
immune system   23, 162
immunoglobulin   28, 138
immunoglobulins A   155
immunoglobulins G   155
immunoglobulins M   155
Impulse Dermotest   127
infections   165
inflammation   8, 173
inflammation mediators   47
inflammatory processes   156
inflammatory rheumatic disease   133
inflammatory rheumatism   201
inflammatory systemic diseases   193
influenza   145
information   19
inosite phosphate   48
inosite triphosphate   19
inspiration   92
insulin shock   169
intestinal colic   196
intestinal flora   178
iodine consumption   132
iodometry   144, 150, 178, 184
iron   61, 160
isodesmosin   66
isolectric point   8
isoionia   19
isoosmia   19
isotonia   19

K
K^+ 51
keratan sulfate   56
kinetic chain   118
kinetic energy   74

L
Lambliasis   195
laminin   19, 69, 72
larynx carcinoma   173
Lathryogen   66
LDL   28, 29
leukocytes   20, 30, 31, 33, 34, 144, 155
leukocytolysis   38, 40
leukolysis   32, 38, 41, 138
leukotriens   29
lipoprotein   28
liquid crystals   52
liquid-crystaline water   73, 76
lung process   89
lymph extract   174
lymphatics   8, 16
lymphocytes   33, 34, 36, 170
lymphocytosis   169
lymphokins   31
lysine   61

M
macrophages   20, 47, 164
magnetic fields   107
manganese   160
mannose   69
mast cells   20, 46
measles   172
mesenchymal tissue   73
mesenchyme   174
metallothionine   161
micro- and macroangiopathies   28
microfibrils   66
microorganisms   151, 200
midbrain-hypophysis   184
migration   165
minerals   177, 193
mitochondria   43
model   15
molecular rhythm   44
monocyte factor   34, 167, 169, 190
monocytes   138
MS   171, 191, 201

multiple sclerosis 133, 171
myelin 27
myocardial infarction 182

N
N-acetyl-galactosamine 55
N-acetylglucosamine 46, 69
N-glycosidic bindings 58, 60
Na^+ 51
nervous system 15
neural therapy 128, 132
neurotransmitter 194
Newton 7
Newtonian systems 76
nucleic acids 41

O
O-glycosidic bindings 56, 60
oligosaccharide 57
open-energy systems 76, 143
opsonin 71
orthostasis 121
oscillation 84, 107
oscillatory behaviour 87
ossification 62
oxygen 26, 61
oxygen treatment 187
oxyhemoglobin 142, 156, 174
oxytalan 67

P
palpation 125
PAPS 55
Paracelsus 17, 76
PCP 202
penicillin 36, 38, 39
Permeability Pathology 16
PG/GAGs 19, 20
PGs 27, 58, 61
physiological lysis 30
piezoelectrical power 64
piezoelectrical properties 107
pituitary-adrenal axis 202
pituitary-adrenal function 163
platelet factor 4 47
polarization 105
polyanions 59
polyarthritis 162
polymerization 27
polysaccharide 28
potential difference 105

potential energy 74
precellular evolution 77
pre-collagen 61
proline 61
prostaglandins 29
proteoglycans 19, 24, 27, 114
proteolytic enzymes 29
protocollagen 66
protozoonoses 177
psychoneuroimmunology 23
puncture reaction 133

Q
quantum chemistry 77

R
radiation 35
radicals 27
receptive field 96
receptors 59
reference zone 102
regulation 83
regulator 85
regulatory blockade 127
regulatory disintegration 117
regulatory paralysis 150
regulatory therapy 98
rehabilitation medicine 89
remote disturbance 109
renal function 196
renal glomeruli 51
repolarization 198
RES 40, 174
resonance reaction 87
respiration 93
rheography 140
rheological changes 20
rheumatism 171
rhombo-mesencephalic control system 104
rhythmogenesis 124
RNA 20, 26, 47, 62, 161, 194
RNA polymerases 172
rotation symmetry 65
rubella 172

S
scars 160, 180
Schelling 78
Schiff's base 66
second messengers 43

secondary stress   109
segmental-regulatory complex   99, 103
selenium   160
seminoma   173
sensory-motor control   95
shock   71, 147, 152, 154, 167, 189
sialinic acid   59, 69
side-differences   158
signal peptides   61
skin   180, 183
sleep-wake rhythm   44
slow viruses   193
sol   111
somatomotor reflexes   104
spinal segments   95
spirometric tests   91
starch   77
stoerfeld   90
stress   89, 168
structural glycoproteins   24
structure breakers   54
structure makers   54
sugar polymers   24
sugar surface film   14
superoxide dysmutase   26
symbiotics   176, 191
synapse   71

T
T lymphocytes   172
T-cell   161, 171
telopeptides   62
thermodiagnosis   125
thoracic spine   94
thrombus   72
tissue hormones   31
toxins   177, 198
toxoplasmosis   172
trace elements   177, 193
transcription   20
transit route   16
transmitter function   15
trigger-points   45
Trisomia 21   28

tropocollagen   63, 65
tropoelastin   66
tuberculosis   89
tumor cells   49
tumor matrix vesicles   42
tumors   13, 202
type I collagen   63, 64
type II collagen   63
type III collagen   63, 67
type IV collagen   63
type V collagen   63

U
UDP   55
ulcerative colitis   133, 201
uric acid   28
uronic acids   45
UV irridation   186

V
vaccine   151
vegetative nerve fibers   20
vegetative-nervous structure   8
vertebra   94
vessel-nerve bundles   45
Virchow   7, 13
visceromotor reflexes   104
viscoelasticity   68
vitamin A   26, 196
vitamin B   196
vitamin C   33, 51
vitamin E   26
vitamins   177, 193

W
Waalsian charges   74
water   46, 52, 53, 73

X
x-rays   183

Z
zinc   160